Those Adventurous Winters

By

Lola Neeley

ISBN: 1-4107-4738-7 (e-book)
ISBN: 1-4107-4739-5 (Paperback)

Library of Congress Control Number: 2003092662

This book is printed on acid free paper.

Printed in the United States of America
Bloomington, IN

1stBooks - rev. 06/07/03

TABLE OF CONTENTS

DEDICATION

In memory of my beloved parents, Jake and Nell McCurry.

To
Judith
Thanks
Lola Neeley
Ph
457 3346

PREFACE

KANSAS TERRITORY 1900's

THOSE ADVENTUREOUS WINTER'S

16 year old, Bob Winter, son of Jacob and Abby Winter, left home to see the world. He was tired of being on the family farm where he, his six brothers, five sisters and parents lived in mostly happy pandemonium.

Bob joined up with some young men who like himself, were hell bent on adventure, rustling a few cattle only to be chased by a posse. His friends were caught and hanged as Bob watched from a plum thicket where his horse had thrown him before it had run off.

Bob, afraid the posse was still looking for him and afraid he would receive the same punishment as his friends, kept to a trail that led away from the direction of the posse.

After living by his wits, experiencing hunger, cold and danger and with the aide of an old mountain man, he survived. He returned to his family near his 18th birthday.

Papa Winter was the head of the family and ran a strict system of what each member of the family's duties were and which chore was performed at what time. Everyone had to work every day to feed the family of 14.

As each son became of an age to take over a job held by an employee, the employee was let go and the son knew he was now responsible and did his duty without hesitation or argument.

The five hundred acres of farm and pasture land for their large dairy herd, which was milked morning and night by hand, kept every family member occupied. In the summer, the two older girls helped with the milking, allowing the boys to get into the field at daybreak where they worked until dark every day except Sunday during harvest time.

Jenny, the eldest daughter was allowed to go to London to study dress design, which she had dreamed of all her life. She spent years of study at Arlton's, a fashion school and manufacturer of fine clothes and materials coveted by women everywhere. That is where she met, fell in love with and married James Arlton, the son of Lady Arlton, the head of Arlton Designs.

Each of the Winter boys always wanted to see over the next hill.

Weldon, Weld for short, was more eager than the rest. Traveling from Kansas to California by horse and boxcar, on the very new steam locomotives when available.

After a year he continued his travels to London then to Paris, experiencing life as he had never known it.

Women chased after both Weld and Bob, but neither was ready to settle down. Weld loved the ladies but would never take advantage of a good girl, nor would any of the Winter men. They would dance and do a little petting, but when it came to calming their biological urges, they chose women that had no interest in anything more than sexual pleasure. All the Winter men were experts in the art of lovemaking.

Henry and Jack followed Weld's lead and went to London, citing the need to see their sister. Jack ended up in Paris, posing for the same artist that had sculpted a life-sized nude of Weld and he visited some of the same establishments Weld had visited. They both ended up having relations with the same well-known lady of the night. Jack made many friends before going back to London, where he decided to stay and work for his sister.

As he was 1/3 owner of the Bar-X-Z, Weld taught Bob everything about caring for the ranch before he took off to wander around and ended up visiting the home farm in Kansas. While Weld was at the farm, Jacob, his Father, was kicked in the head by a stallion and died. Jacob's wife Abby, died just hours later. They had been deeply in love their entire lives and she just could not face life without her beloved husband. Three of the Winter men were married by then, having farms and families of their own. They needed money to build and to plant crops. The will was read, giving information on deeds, monies and requesting the care of the three smaller daughters. The surviving family members were to decide whether to keep or to sell the farm, dividing the funds between themselves. Long tedious preparations and decisions over how to manage everything fairly, took the best part of a year. There were and still are stong love matches, romances and dalliances by the Winter men, but always as gentlemen. The farm is still in the Winter family, where the influence of Jacob and Abby Winter's strong family creed still guide the new generations.

CHAPTER 1

Bob lay as low as he could behind a Wild Plum thicket, trying to keep the posse from locating him. They were busy throwing two ropes across a limb on a huge Elm tree, makin' ready to hang his best friends for cattle russlin'.

This was Bob's third time out takin' cattle that did not belong to him. Until now no one had even chased them. He had felt safe. They had planned each job meticulously. Nothing could possibly go wrong.

He was just eight days from turning eighteen and was going to die within the next few minutes unless he could stay hidden well enough and long enough to evade this posse.

Bob hid his face and closed his eyes as he heard the snap of the ropes. He knew his friends were dead.

The posse rode back toward town while Bob still lay behind the Plum thicket. His legs would not stop trembling and his stomach was so upset he would have puked if he had, had anything in it. As it was it just surged in dry heaves.

He had no horse. It had bolted and run away which had probably saved his life. Now all he had was Shank's Mare to get far from here in these Missouri hills. How he longed for home and family back in Kansas.

He had left the farm to see the world when he was sixteen and was doing all right until he had met Jim and Trey. They had spoken of easy money and great adventures' and he had joined them. Now see where he was, a reward on his head and stuck.

Bob waited until dark and headed away from town. He didn't want to run into that posse.

His feet were blistered and his heels were running pus by next day. He carried his boots which were mostly worn out. Reaching a creek, he sat and soaked his tender feet in the cold water. The swelling went down some and the burning was almost gone.

Bob was able to catch a couple of frogs, hitting them with rocks. He also caught a baby rabbit which he cooked over a fire on a stick. He strained water through his neckerchief into his mouth. He didn't want to take a chance on swallowing a water snake as his father had when he was young. Bob had heard that story many times.

It was too hot to walk on sore feet so he decided to take a nap. He sat with his back against a tree, pulled his hat down over his face and went to sleep. It was dark when he woke. There was no moon. He could not see an inch in front of himself.

"Well I might just as well go back to sleep," he said to himself. "My feet need more healing time anyway."

He thought he was dreaming. Someone was jabbing him in the side with the toe of a boot. Bob quickly opened his eyes and looked up into the smiling face of a huge bearded man.

"Watcha doin' here Sonny? Where's yur hoss and why are yuh barefeeted?"

"I'm here because some Jack of Napes stoled my hoss and I'm barefoot because I had tuh walk twenty miles more or less."

"Wal Sonny, come wid me. We can have a bite and yuh can ride my mule. He ain't loaded heavy."

'Where are yuh goin?" Bob inquired.

"Wat difference do it make? Yuh cain't stay here."

"Nope. I guess yer right. It don't matter where I'm goin'. What's yer name?" Bob asked the big man.

"Oh, jest call me Sam. Wat's yern?"

Bob almost gave his real name, but remembered the reward posters and said "Jim."

They had come upon an open cave like place, hidden behind some trees and huge boulders. The big man had gingerly woven his way between the rocks and trees to the cave. If you didn't know there was a cave around here you could never have found it except by accident.

Inside the cave was a large room area where many cured hides were stacked. There were also blankets, a tin pail, three rusty tin plates, a variety of hunting knives and several whittled forks and spoons. In the back of the cave was a ring of rocks where Sam did his cooking over a fire. Above the fire ring was an opening where smoke could escape.

Sam explained, "Nivver light a far in day light. The smoke can be seen from a long way off."

Bob didn't ask why Sam didn't want anyone to see the smoke, but it was good for him as well.

About fifteen feet west of the cave opening was a rock shelf that served as a barn for Sam's hoss and mule. It was well hidden, as was the cave.

Sam would go out everyday and bring back meat, wild greens, roots and berries. A tiny stream of water ran down the rocks just to the right of the entrance of the cave, affording them plenty of fresh water to drink, cook and bathe with. The only thing they really needed was a couple of pots to cook in.

Sam said. "One of dese days, I gond ta fine a campsite wid no body der and git a pot fer cookin'."

Each of them had cured hides to sleep on and blankets to cover up with.

Bob figured Sam had been out of contact with any human beings for a very long time. His clothes were tattered, but clean. He had made Bob and himself moccasins out of hides and had fashioned panchos as well. He had used dried strips of skin to sew the hides together using a Turkey rib bone as a needle.

They often fished in the creek about a mile away. Sam was very adept at catching Trout and Bass. Bob however, didn't quite get the hang of noodling for fish under rocks or in grassy patches next to the bank where Bass like to hide.

The moccasins had allowed Bob's feet to heal. He had gotten used to feeling pebbles underfoot through the soles of his shoes. At first it had felt as if they were puncturing his feet but now he was fine with the soft soles and it was hard to track a foot shod in a moccasin.

Sam had never asked Bob anything about his private life before they had met, nor had Bob ask Sam anything. Neither of them offered any information to the other.

It was mid summer and Bob knew he had to start for his home in Kansas soon. If he waited much longer the weather would be too cold to travel and he had a long way to go. He hated to leave Sam but he had learned his lesson well. If he ever got back to kith and kin he would never stray again. Bob told Sam it was time for him to leave. He told him where his home was and how far it was. He explained how cold it got in the fall and winter in the states he had to cross.

"Well Sonny, yuh cain't walk all dat fur. Yer gond ta need a hoss. Duz yuh got eny money?" Sam asked.

"I have about four dollars," Bob said.

"Yuh cain't buy no hoss wid dat," Sam stated holding out a small leather bag of gold coins. "Here yuh are Sonny."

"Oh Sam, I cain't take yer money. Yuh will need it yer self."

"Don'cha worry nun 'bout me. I know whar thar is a plenty more whar that comed frum. 'Cides, wat can I buy wid it out cher?" Sam came back.

Bob gave Sam his address and told him, "Come see me. Yer welcome any time."

"Sonny, I jest might do dat one day."

****

CHAPTER 2

Bob made it to a small ranch where he bought a good horse and saddle. He paid the rancher from his pouch and got on his way.

The rancher had told him the horse's name was Socks, due to the four white socks he was marked with. He rode slowly, letting Socks choose his gait. They had a long way to go and plenty of time to become acquainted.

In early Fall Bob had to stop in a town to get Socks some new shoes and to give both of them a chance to rest up a bit. The bill of sale for Socks was made out to Jim Smith. If anyone needed proof of who he was, he could use this document as identification.

The first day and night in town Bob spent in bed. The following day he walked over to "Pa's Eatin' House" and ate the first real meal he had, had in months and drank three cups of coffee.

He checked on Socks and found he had been shod and had been well fed. "I'll pick him up early in the morning," Bob told the Smithy. "Do yuh want me tuh pay yuh now, or before I leave?"

"When yuh pick 'im up is fine," the Smithy smiled.

Daylight was just beginning to break when Bob finished his breakfast and had Pa, to sack him up some food for the road. He had wandered down to the Smithy's, paid him and was on his way again. Socks, was rested and ready to go but Bob held him at a slow gait. They weren't goin far today, just outside of town there was a nice clear water creek, where he could get his laundry cleaned up and dried on the bushes in the warm sunshine of the day. He still had hundreds of miles to go and he wanted everything clean.

Bob had seen two posters tacked on trees since he had left Sam. Neither one was for him but he kept his eyes peeled.

He had purchased new clothing, shaved his beard off and cut his hair as well. He really didn't look like the sixteen year old that had run with a gang of cattle thieves.

Bob made camp a mile or so outside of town. He didn't want to come in contact with anyone, especially some Drunked up Cowhand. He couldn't afford any kind of conflict that could bring the sheriff around.

He tethered Socks close to where he would put his bedroll after he had finished with his laundry. He bedded down around dusk having finished his domestic chores and had eaten his food that Pa had fixed. He slept at once.

It must have been around midnight when people speaking in hushed tones wakened him.

He could only make out part of what was being said but he sure didn't like the part he heard. The tall thin man was saying, "Make sure to be at the bank when they first open the door. Slip in and lock the door from the inside. Wait till the banker opens the safe, cold-cock him with yer gun and scoop all the money into this," he said handing him a small sack. The two then rode slowly toward town.

Bob didn't know what to do. He knew he had to be far from there long before morning but what to do about the planned bank robbery!

He decided to use the back of an envelope he had picked up at the Rooming House, to write a warning to the sheriff. How to get it to him was the problem.

He figured he'd take the envelope to Pa's Eatin' Place and try to leave it in a spot where it couldn't be missed. But how could he know if Pa may be in on the robbery him self.

The Blacksmith's, that's where he would take the note. The Smithy got up early, and if he was involved, "Well, too bad," Bob thought. "It's the best I can do."

At one thirty in the morning Bob knocked on the Smithy's door leaving the note wedged in a crack in the door. He watched from across the street in the shadows of the Rooming House. Just as soon as he saw the Smithy start down the street toward the jail, he took off, riding slowly and quietly.

Bob never did hear a word about what, if anything had happened but his conscience was clear.

"Hey feller, your hoss is loose." He heard someone saying. He looked up and sure enough, Socks had some how slipped his hobble and had strayed off.

"Thanks, I sure appreciate yer tellin' me. I was just takin' myself a little siesta and lettin' my hoss graze."

Bob wasn't quite sure what state he was in, so he asked, "Where am I? I think I'm kinda lost."

"Yer in Clayton Arkansas or will be when yuh git over that hill" he said pointing west.

Home was getting closer. He was about four hundred miles from there and a good thing it was. It had been getting mighty cold at night. He was glad Sam had insisted that he take the pancho and a fine fur robe for his shoulders.

Bob rode into town taking in the different places of business, the sheriff's jail and the saloon. He had shied away from saloons up to now, trying not to meet up with any one he might have known before or some joker wanting to fight.

Bob wasn't a fighter but he wasn't afraid either, except for the sheriff. It had been so long since he had been around anyone he thought he would take a chance. He had forgotten how loud it was in saloons. With him being alone for so long, it probably sounded even louder to him.

"Anyone here want a job ridin' shotgun on the stage? Ya hafta be a good shot and ready ta fight if need be."

A tall thin man and a smaller fella came forward and offered to take the job. Bob remembered that voice and a tall man and a shorter one. They had been the two plannin' the bank job.

No way could Bob be on the road when this was to take place. "Just how was he goin' tuh get this information tuh the right people in time tuh stop it?" he wondered.

He took a room at the only spot in town that afforded a place to sleep. Again he fashioned a note still not knowing how or who to get it to. He walked the street from one end to the other. He finally decided to take the chance at the stage office. He walked in and asked what time the next stage would leave and was told in about two hours. When the clerk turned away for a moment he tossed the note onto the desk and walked to a small eating place he had seen. He ordered a steak, potatoes and eggs and kept his eye on the stage office.

He had an unobstructed view of the office from where he sat eating waiting to see some kind of movement from the clerk or driver. It was nearly an hour before the clerk ran out the office door showing the driver a piece of paper. The driver became excited and rushed over to the sheriff's office. Now there was a lot of movement going on.

Bob smiled. "What a law abiding citizen I have become."

He guessed it was all right for him to move on now. Socks was getting fed and curried, watered and rubbed down but should be about ready to go now.

Bob paid the man and bought a feedbag full of grain for Socks. In places grass was very sparse now. He was now in Kansas but it was still almost two hundred miles to his folk's farm.

Bob had bought himself some gloves at his last stop. He had also bought some heavy socks and long johns, two pair of each. He would probably have to put all of them on at once before he made it home. He had also gotten Socks a full size horse blanket.

Snow was falling right smart now. Bob said to himself, "It must be about Halloween time." Oh what he would give to be at the holiday feast. His mouth watered remembering the pies, ham, sweet potatoes and corn pudding. Ummm.

It was December sixteenth and Bob would soon be home when all hell broke loose. A man of perhaps one hundred eighty pounds was beating, kicking and stomping a hapless little man senseless. No one was interfering. Bob asked "Why?"

"Everyone is afraid of Tom Port. He would kill anyone who tried to help poor Mr. Moore."

"Well he's damn sure gond to kill that man if no one stops him!" Bob said. "Oh hell," he thought as he lifted his gun from his holster and struck the big man across the temple. The big man fell across Mr. Moore and Bob rolled him off the smaller man.

Everyone gasped! "Oh Lordy, there is hell to pay now. Feller yuh don't know what yuh have done. He will kill ya."

"I surely hope not but no way could I stand by and watch a man be murdered," Bob said.

The sheriff came slowly down the street. Someone had reported that Tom Port was killing Mr. Moore. The sheriff didn't want any part of Tom Port. No one would go up against Tom.

"What's takin' place?" asked the sheriff, seeing both men lying in the street.

"I guess I'm the one yer askin' 'bout," Bob said.

"Yuh mean yuh did this to Tom?"

"Well, I reckon so. I just couldn't see a man stomping a helpless unconscious person, so I slapped him across the temple with my gun."

"Young fella, yuh had better be on yur way. Git on down the road, cuz Tom's gond tuh come after yuh soons he wakes up."

"Are yuh gond tuh keep him off these town's people? They tell me if I'm not around, he will finish off Mr. Moore and probly beat half the men in town tuh death."

The sheriff looked away then back at Bob. "Yuh reckon yuh could hang around a couple of days tuh help me with 'im?"

"Cain't yuh just put him in jail a couple of days till he cools down?"

"Nope, I'd hafta let 'im go sooner or later and I'd have the same problem I have now."

"Swear me in as deputy. I'll see what can be done," Bob said. They carried Tom to jail and got him on the cot just as he was coming to. They hurried out of the cell and locked the door leaving the building. They didn't want to listen to him yell and threaten.

Dr. Marks was bending over Mr. Moore in the street.

"How is he?" Bob asked.

"Far as I can tell here, he has some broken ribs and his left arm is broken. He is spitting up blood, so he has some internal bleeding. He isn't fully conscious and he doesn't respond to anything. He may not make it," the doctor said.

Bob looked at the sheriff and inquired. "Yuh just allow a man tuh do this kinda thing when he feels like it?" The sheriff shrugged and looked away.

Bob went back to the jail where Tom was tearing everything in the cell to pieces. He was cussing every breath he took and swearing to kill every son of a bitch, when he got out.

"Yuh might do that, but yuh may never git out if Mr. Moore dies."

"Dies? What do yuh mean die? He ain't hurt. I just roughed him up a little fer bumping in ter me at the bank. The little four eyed bastard orta watch where he's goin."

"Well Tom, the Doctor says he may not make it. He's all broke up inside as well as outside."

"Now! Now! Wait jest a minute. I ain't no killer. I jest got a quick temper."

"Yuh sure do that all right. Yuh let yur temper rule yuh and take out all yur unhappiness on innocent people. Further more, yur goin' tuh pay fer all that stuff yuh tore up in there or yuh ain't gettin' no food or different stuff to sleep or sit on!"

Tom was plum flabbergasted. No one ever talked to him like this kid was doing, since his mother used to when she put him over her knee when he was just a kid.

"What are yuh gond tuh do when I git outta here so's I can git tuh yuh?"

"Like I told yuh, I hope that don't happen but if it does, yuh better come ready tuh die cause I aim tuh kill yuh. There just ain't no place in this world fer people like yuh. Yuh bring nuthin' but unhappiness and pain tuh everyone yuh come into contact with."

Tom was very quiet. He lay on the mattress on the floor thinking. All night he thought and didn't cause any more trouble of any kind. He said a little prayer, telling God, "If yuh will please let Mr. Moore live and git well, I'll never raise a hand to another human being as long as I live."

Bob brought Tom some breakfast at nine a.m. Tom accepted it silently. "How's Mr. Moore?" he asked Bob.

"The Doctor says he is gond tuh make it but will be laid up fer maybe six months. The little man is worried about his family. He cain't work and he is the only bread winner for his wife and five younguns."

Tom handed Bob his plate. "Tell Moore not tuh fret. I'll see that his family and him are taken care of."

Bob nodded.

"Sheriff, I'll be leavin' in the mornin'. I've got tuh get home tuh my family, hopefully fer Christmas," Bob said.

"Hey, wait a minute. Yuh said yuh would stay and help me handle Tom," said the sheriff.

"Yuh won't need any help. He's gond tuh be fine and so is Mr. Moore's family. Bob stated.

"How can yuh say a thing like that?" asked the sheriff.

"Oh, a little birdie told me. Just believe me. He won't cause no more problems fer yuh or anyone else.

Bob rode into his Father's drive lane at two p.m. on December twenty fourth, nineteen o five.

"Son? My son Bob?" his mother cried. She hardly recognized him.

He had changed so much since she had last seen him. "Oh my baby! My baby! We all thought you were dead. We heard you had been hanged in Missouri Territory almost three years ago."

"Well here I am. I'm very alive and I'm starved. I need tuh get outta all these clothes and have a bath. My horse needs taken care of first so I'll see yuh in a little while."

"Son, let the boys tend to your horse. They will take good care of him. Come I will have a tub of warm water and soap sent up to your old room and some clean clothes too."

"Its so good tuh be home. I'll never run away again," Bob promised.

"Oh son, it has been such a sad time believing you were dead. Where have you been all these years? You left here a boy but you've come back a man," she cried.

"I'll tell yuh all about it but let's wait until we are all together. I do need that bath now!" he assured her.

Bob just wanted to stay in the tub and never get out it felt so wonderful and smelled so good. “Mama must have put some of her ‘Rose Water’ that she makes every summer, into the bath water,” he thought.

The fireplace crackled and danced, making the room warm and cozy. Finally however he got out of the tub and rubbed himself dry. The clothes his mother had left laid out on the bed were all nicely ironed. This was something he had not experienced since he had left home.

Bob was wondering if he should tell all. He sure didn’t want it to get out about the cattle rustling, him being part of it. If he didn’t tell it, how could he explain about his being on the run for such a long time and how about the posters and the folks being told he had been hanged?

He could smell food cooking and hear voices from downstairs. Well, he would just have to go face the music and play it by ear.

Bob had six brothers older than he and two older sisters. There were also three younger sisters, Mildred eight, Harriet five and little

Rosie four. They had all been very young when Bob had left and none of them remembered him. The two older sisters were Jenny and Raye. Of the boys Jeremy was the eldest followed by Carl and Frank, Henry, Weldon and Jackson. No one ever dared call 'Weldon', Weldon. He was "Weld" and could kick anyone's behind that said otherwise. All the Winter boys were rough and ready but not a one was a trouble maker. They all attended to their own business but if you ever thought you could take advantage of any one of them you better think again.

Mr. Winter their Father, was as big and strong as the boys with the same attitude and behavior. He still had a heavy shock of red hair with no grey showing anyplace. His face was smooth and free of lines but he had a spattering of freckles as did all the boys except for Bob, who had dark brown hair like his mother's. None of the girls had freckles, except little Rosie. The two older girl's hair was neither red nor brown, but somewhere in between.

Mother Abby was still a very handsome woman and after twelve younguns still had a figure that would make a young woman jealous.

Abby never primped or powdered. She had a peaches and cream complexion that needed no enhancements.

Jacob had married Abby when he was twenty and she was just eighteen. Right away they started a family intending on having four or five children, but some how the babies just kept coming. Now at age fifty and twelve younguns later he and Abby were still as much in love as ever. They still made mad passionate love everyday, their ardor never having waned. Now with no worry of Abby becoming pregnant again life was wonderful. Bob was home the farm was producing well and was paid for. There was money enough for everything they needed and he had started paying the boys regular salaries three years ago.

Every one of the boys banked two thirds of their salaries each month building up a nest egg for the time they married and left home. All of them hired out when every thing was finished at the farm. They banked their wages from those jobs as well. All were home schooled for the most part. Abby had taught them every day. She took three hours daily to give school lessons year round except for Sundays. No one was required to do anything on Sundays except milk twice a day and throw feed to the animals. There was no way around that. Cows must be milked twice a day and fed at each milking.

The kitchen was huge. It sported a really big six lid range from France with an oven large enough to accommodate a thirty six biscuit sized pan. The boys young and growing put the food away at the rate of starving race horses. Large glasses of milk which were refilled two or three time each meal grits, eggs and slabs of salt pork or bacon for breakfast and supper at night was like cooking for a harvest crew. Potatoes fried, mashed, baked or boiled, brown beans, greens and corn bread and fruit and the ever present milk along with cheese and clabber were available for those who liked it. They ate at the same time every day, six a.m. and six p.m. No noon meal except through harvest when it was so hot and the men needed their strength.

Everyone sat around the four leaf table in the dining area eager to hear all about Bob's adventures.

"Where ya been son?" Jacob asked. "What happened about that hanging we heard about?"

"I left here and bummed my way through Kansas, Missouri, Arkansas and Indiana and back to Missouri, where I met a couple of fellers wantin' tuh have some fun and make a lot of money easy, they said. Me lookin' fer adventure joined up with Jim and Trey who had some experience russlin' and I found it fun and exciting. I stood lookout while the other two gathered up half a dozen or so cattle and turned them over to another feller to sell. We weren't getting' rich but we were having a lot of fun."

"But Bob," his mother intervened, "You were not raise to take other folks property."

"I know Mama but remember, I was only sixteen and a half and I never gave a thought as tuh how it might affect the ranchers," Bob explained.

He told them all about how he had escaped detection and of his meeting up with Sam. He told about Sam giving him the pouch of gold coins and how Sam had said he knew where there was plenty more where that came from.

"I still have close to five hundred dollars left in the pouch," Bob told them.

He didn't leave out a thing that had happened on his way home. He even included his short stint as deputy and the trouble with Tom Post.

****

CHAPTER 3

The eldest sister Genevieve, Jenny for short, had been keeping company with one of the Haskin boys for about a year now. He was urging her to set a date but she just wasn't sure she was ready for marriage at eighteen. She had never been further then twenty miles from the farm. She had only met three boys other than her brothers in her whole life. Jenny often felt she was not meant to be a farmer's wife. She dreamed of far away places and handsome young men on big white horses carrying her off to his castle in England or Spain or some other romantic hide away. A place where Maidens dressed in bright costumes waited on them and entertained them.

She didn't dare voice these thoughts to anyone else. Not even her sisters or her Mother. They would laugh and hoorah her saying how silly she was. Never the less she still dreamed her dreams.

Jenny was a great seamstress. She copied patterns out of magazines and papers her parents had delivered every month to their home. She devoured every printed word that came into view. She looked longingly at stone mansions and castles in foreign lands. "I just know that's where I belong," she would tell herself.

Patrick Haskin called on Jenny on Saturday afternoon. They went for a walk. Pat held her hand and said, "I love you Jenny, I need you. When are you going to set the date?"

Jenny turned to Pat with tears in her eyes. "Pat, I just cannot marry you. I just don't want to be married. I'm going to England to be a seamstress. I want to design beautiful clothes for famous people. Daddy has agreed to send me to London. If I cannot make it there, I'll have to come back and find a way to make a living on my own."

Pat did not say a word. He turned on his heel got on his horse and rode quite fast down the lane to the road.

The trip overseas was agony for Jenny. She was seasick most of the voyage. While the other passengers gathered on deck to enjoy the sea air and the sun Jenny was hanging her head over the rail heaving.

She did meet a nice looking and acting man. He was from London. He was going home after a two month visit to his mother in America. He was eager to get back to his home.

"America's wild country isn't my cup of tea," he told Jenny.

"Jenny confided in Paul, (that was the man's name) that she was going to London to learn dress design from Arlton's of London.

"Oh yes, I know James Arlton. He belongs to the same club as I. Would you like me to introduce you?"

"Would you?" she asked. I don't know a soul there, except for you," she smiled. "Isn't it a real coincidence my meeting you and you knowing a relative of Arltons?"

"Oh he is not just a relative! He is the eldest son of Peggy Arlton, the head of Arlton's."

"They are really nice people! You wouldn't think they were wealthy. Not stuck up at all," he told Jenny, grinning.

"When we get to London would you care to dine with me, Miss Jenny?"

"Well, I don't really know you, er, Paul. I have been warned to keep my character in good stead if I ever intend to make it anywhere."

"Oh I can fix that!" Paul said smiling.

Soon he returned to the deck, bringing the ship's Captain to where she sat. "Captain, would you please introduce me to Miss Winter and tell her what a nice fellow I am." he laughed.

Gladly the Captain agreed. "Miss Winter may I present Mr. Paul Sims, from London? Mr. Sims, may I present Miss Jenny Winter from Kansas, in America?"

"Now see! That was easy enough, wasn't it?" he laughed again.

"Yes I'll dine with you," she said, "and thanks so much."

When the ship docked there was a scramble everyone trying to go ashore at once, except Jenny and Paul.

Paul had told her, "Let's just wait until almost everyone else has gone ashore. Do you have a place to stay, some arrangements?" he inquired of her.

"No I haven't. Daddy said to ask the Captain to recommend a small hotel in a safe district that I can afford. Would you know of such a place, Mr. Sims?"

"As a matter of fact, I do. We can take a Tram from here. It is only a short way."

Jenny was a little apprehensive. After all, he was a perfect stranger to her.

Paul noticed her hesitancy and called the Captain over. "Captain, can you tell Miss Winter where she might locate an affordable small hotel or rooming house in a safe area in London?"

Paul waited until the Captain had a moment to think. "Oh yes, there is a small place called "The Shakes." It is a nice little place where you can get meals if you care to, and they have a guard on duty to insure no unwanted person will drop in."

"Exactly!" Paul agreed. "Just where I was telling Jenny to visit, at least until she gets to know her way around."

Paul took Jenny to a quaint little place that specialized in seafood. He ordered for both of them, family style. They had platters of shrimp, crab, octopus, scallops, lobster and plenty of salad.

London was foggy so much of the time very different from Kansas. Jenny found the weather depressing and it affected her artistic ability to design.

Arlton's had given her free reign after hours, to create on her own. She was learning so much and loved every moment of it. It was just the weather and the homesickness that made her feel so alone, so lost.

Paul Sims invited her out on the average of twice a week. He was good company and Jenny really liked him but she had little free time with studies and working up designs of her own.

She had not met James Arlton yet but was looking forward to it. She got the impression that he was a bit of a man about town.

Jenny wrote long letters home to her family and had received two letters. One was from her mother and one from her sister Raye who was just one year younger than her self. Daddy and all her brothers sent their love. Oh how she missed them, all of them.

It was Christmas again, nineteen o six. Just one year had passed since Jenny's youngest brother had returned from his near fatal adventure. She remembered how happy they had all been to have him home, safe and in good health. She wondered if any of them missed her as much as she missed them.

There was no snow in London but the grey weather chilled her to the bone. She didn't know if it ever snowed in London or not but she hoped it would.

A package was delivered to the hotel for her. It was from her family. When she opened it she cried. There were all kinds of homemade candies like the ones Mama always made for Christmas. There were the candies and an assortment of jams and jellies, as well as two beautiful Tortoise Shell combs for her hair. Now she really was lonesome.

Paul came by and insisted she let him take her to dinner and later to the "Nutcracker" at the new theatre that Arlton's had donated to the city.

She was really glad she had accepted the invitation. The food was delicious, although nothing like the food served at home. She had enjoyed the Nutcracker immensely and it was a new experience for her.

Paul returned her to her room at The Shakes about ten thirty p.m. "It is still early," Paul said. "Could we sit in the lobby and talk?"

"Oh Paul you have been so nice to me and I would really love to but I cannot. I have an early sitting, very early, for a dress I am making!" Jenny exclaimed.

"Another time then," he smiled. Jenny agreed, wondering why Paul wasn't celebrating Christmas with his family.

Jenny had fashioned a ball gown of wine colored velvet, with crystal beads sewn onto the neckline and down the back opening. The beads glittered next to the wine velvet and the richness of the fabric was really beautiful.

On January eighth, nineteen o seven, Jenny presented her first design at Arlton's, and got rave reviews. She was so excited and needed someone to celebrate with, only there was no one. Jenny had no idea where Paul lived and no way to contact him. He was the only person she knew outside the people she worked with and they were not social acquaintances.

It was six p.m. when Paul showed up and congratulated her on her success. "How did you know?" she asked.

"James told me," he said. "I had spoken of you many times to him and he remembered when the notices came out at the shop. From what I hear everyone is excited about your design."

Jenny was so happy she could hardly say a word. "I must write my family!" she said.

"I'm sure they will be very proud of you," Paul stated. "I'm meeting James for drinks at his home, will you join us?" Paul inquired.

"Are you sure Mr. Arlton would want me there? As of yet, we have never met." Jenny stated.

"As a matter of fact he asked me to bring you," Paul explained.

When they climbed into Paul's Brougham and headed for James Arlton's home, Jenny suddenly felt as though she should turn back and not continue to Mr. Arlton's.

The countryside was beautiful. There were very few estates but all were grand and huge, with well kept grounds.

When they came abreast of a huge castle, Paul pointed and said, "This is where I live."

Jenny was sure he was fooling and said as much.

"No, I'm telling the truth," he said. "Where did you think I might live?"

She was flustered. "Well, I just supposed you lived somewhere in a regular house, or a flat," she sighed.

Some three miles further Paul turned into a gated estate so large it looked like the castles she had read about while growing up. She expected at any moment to see Knights on white horses appear from the wooded area that was surrounding the castle. Jenny was gripping the side of the Brougham she was so excited and nervous. When they reached the large front door two liveried servants stepped forward, bringing a small step for her to alight the Brougham.

"Oh my word," she thought. "Just like my books said."

They entered an area where the ceiling was at least twenty five feet high. The floors were of some kind of polished stone with thick woven rugs placed at intervals. All of them a beautiful floral blue, that seemed to be alive. They sparkled with colors of shaded lighter blues. Jenny was afraid to step on the rugs. They were the most beautiful things she had ever seen.

The walls sported huge framed portraits of people from ages before, by the look of their clothing.

There were three fireplaces in the room with heavy candleholders and scented candles. Furniture polished and shone along the walls with fur covered chairs placed in groups with tables at each fireplace. Statues of the finest marble sat at each entrance off the hall.

They were escorted to an equally opulent room. It was not as large or as high a ceiling as the entry area, but Jenny thought, "We could put our whole farmhouse in this room," she was overwhelmed.

A half dozen people were sitting or standing in front of an ornate fireplace of marble with sculptured animals at either side. The men rose as they entered quietly observing Jenny and Paul.

Paul said to the group. "This is Miss Jenny Winter, from America. Jenny may I present Mr. Horton, Mr. Fallon and Mr. Cort." The men each bowed over her hand and kissed it lightly.

They walked further into the room to where the women sat and Paul presented her to each of them. None of the people she met were Arlton's. No James and no Peggy, her boss.

Jenny looked at Paul questioningly. He just smiled and seated her with the ladies.

Everyone was quite friendly and all knew who she was. They were asking her about her design and where in America did she come from and does she have a family? How does she like London? Does she think she might stay in England? Etc. etc.

The gentlemen were just listening. Paul caught her eye and turned his palms up as if to say, "I'm sorry!"

There was the sound of a door being opened and two people stepped through the opening. Jenny immediately knew Peggy Arlton although she had never seen her before. Her portrait hung in the office at Arlton's, where she attended classes. The man she felt sure was James Arlton.

Everyone rose when they entered, so Jenny did as well.

"Be seated my dears," the clear tones of Peggy Arlton's voice instructed. She was a handsome woman of perhaps sixty, perfect from head to toe. She wore a stunning dress of some kind of material Jenny had never seen. It fit her like a second skin at the top but flowed freely from the waist down. It was a totally different concept from the day's fashions.

"Peg, I'd like to present Miss Winter, your very accomplished student, Jenny Winter. Jenny, please make the acquaintance of my sister Peg."

Jenny nearly fainted. "I'm so pleased to meet you Mrs. Arlton," she managed to get the words out. She then turned to Paul, "Your sister? Why haven't you told me before?"

"It didn't seem important to me," he smiled.

"I'm, I'm sorry Mrs. Arlton. I just don't know what to say."

"Say hello and we will all go into dinner."

The dining room was large enough to seat fifty or more but they were seated at a smaller table for twenty. The flame from the fireplace made the crystal glitter. Candles flickered from all over the room.

When Jenny saw all the different knives and forks and different glasses at each plate she panicked. "Oh my goodness! How will I ever get through all this?" she worried. She had been to several elegant places with Paul to eat but nothing like this.

"I'll just have to do as I have always done when Paul has taken me out. I'll watch Paul and do as he does." Jenny ate very little but felt she handled it with grace and poise.

At first she felt stiff and could not enjoy the conversation but about halfway through the meal, she relaxed.

There were nice people and except for perfect manners, very like the folks at home. Instead of talking about farming and cattle, they spoke of traveling, art shows and who is marrying whom and when.

James was a very strong looking man for an Englishman. Most English men seemed soft to Jenny. None she had met had a callous or a broken fingernail. Always they were nattily dressed and soft spoken.

James had a square jawed rugged look about him. His hair was black and wavy and he looked tan and healthy, which can be difficult in London weather. So far Jenny had seen very few, bright sunny days.

After dinner James cornered her and said, "Paul was right. You are a beauty and better yet you are real. You are not like a lot of women we meet in our circle."

"Thank you Mr. Arlton," Jenny said.

"Not Mr. My name is James."

"Very well, James it is," she smiled.

Before Paul took her home James had invited her to have dinner with him on Friday. For some reason Jenny declined saying, "I'm sorry but I won't have a free moment for at least two weeks." James had looked shocked. He wasn't accustomed to any lady turning him down for any reason.

On the way home, Paul inquired of Jenny, "Did you enjoy yourself?"

"Oh I did, indeed. I liked everyone and hope they liked me."

"I assure you, you made a very good impression, especially on James."

"Yes, he asked me out for dinner for Friday," she said. Paul looked angry or at least Jenny thought he did so she quickly assured him that she had refused the invitation.

Paul looked at her thinking, "This is a rare girl indeed." He said aloud, "That's a first. Every girl would give her eye teeth to be asked out by James Arlton."

"After all, you had escorted me there. I didn't feel it appropriate to make a date with one man while being escorted by another," she said primly.

Paul felt very good. He wasn't in love with Jenny but he felt good having found a woman with morals. His wife had never told the truth in her life, at least not to him. She had shamed him by sleeping with every man she met. Everyone knew and had not told him until he had caught her with one of the stable boys about half her age. He had fired the boy on the spot and told her to pack her things and go.

"Like hell I will!" she said. "I'm here and here I'm staying, so just get used to it!!" She had jumped on her horse and rode as fast as she could get the animal to run. Paul and his horse trainer saw her try to make the jump over the gate. The horse stopped abruptly, throwing her over the gate and breaking her neck.

That was two years earlier. He had never let his guard down again until he had met Jenny and that was just friendship. His only child, a son named Peter, was four now and Paul's pride and joy. He spent many hours of complete happiness with his son and expected to introduce Jenny to Peter, soon.

Jenny was very busy for the next two weeks only able to work in one dinner date with Paul. He told her she was working too hard and needed to get out more. "How about dinner at my home on Saturday?' he invited, she accepted.

Jenny was curious as to how Paul lived in comparison to the Arlton's. She didn't have romantic feelings for Paul but she liked him as a person. As she was with females all week at work, she needed male input in her life.

Jenny had worked until noon on a beaded vest like, accessory she had designed for one of Peggy's friends. Sewing each bead in just the right spot was time consuming, but it was a beautiful piece that could be worn with many different costumes.

She couldn't picture anyone at home ever wearing any of the clothes made here, but she had stitched up some cotton dresses to send back home to her mother and her sister Raye. She had also made dresses for the three younger girls and was working on shirts for Daddy and her brothers. Jenny's poor fingers were sore from numerous needle pricks. She always used thimbles but she couldn't protect all of her fingers and even her thumb was sore.

It wouldn't be long now until the instructional part of her studies, were finished and she would actually be designing and cutting. She was so excited and wanted to shout it to everyone. Except for the letters back home she had only Paul to brag to.

Saturday Paul picked Jenny up at six p.m. They chatted happily all the way to Paul's.

Paul's home was large and beautiful but much, more friendly looking than Mrs. Arlton's place. Everything was rich, rich looking and comfortable. Jenny didn't feel as intimidated as she had at the Arlton's. Perhaps it was because she had already been amazed at the opulence of Arlton's.

Jenny thought to herself, "I don't think I could be happy living in a castle. They are just too impersonal. Even though they are warm enough in the rooms that are occupied they just feel cold, a lack of coziness."

Paul brought Peter downstairs to meet Jenny. He was a sweet little boy not the least bit shy. He crawled right into Jenny's lap and began telling her about his pony and how fast he could go.

"Do you have any children?" he asked Jenny.

"No honey I'm not married, but I have three small sisters that I miss so much."

"Can they come play with me? I have many toys to play with and I'll share."

"Oh I wish they were close enough to visit but they are far away in America."

Peter sighed and said, "I get very lonesome for someone to play with. All of Papa's friends only have old children. Sometimes I get to play with 'Cook's' boy. He is five and we have lots of fun but Papa doesn't know or he might send Cook away."

Jenny looked up at Paul who was frowning. "Oh I'm sure Papa would never do a thing like that. He realizes little boys need playmates."

Later after Peter had been put to bed Paul said, "I never realized Peter might be lonely. I just took it for granted he had everything he needed and someone in attendance every moment."

"Children need people their own age to play with," Jenny said. "I cannot imagine how I would have coped without my large family to turn to."

"I'm going to have to do some thinking on this," Paul stated.

****

CHAPTER 4

Bob had his twentieth birthday the same day Jeremy told everyone, “Me and Carley Fauche will be getting’ hitched in May.”

Everyone was caught off guard. None had any inkling that Jerry was seriously courting anyone.

“Ya sure have been tight lipped ‘bout this,” Carl said.

“Yeah, what’s the story? Whyn’t ya ever mention ya was sweet on Carley?”

“Becuz I didn’t want you boys razzin’ me, like ya are right now.” Jerry yelled at them.

They all laughed and grabbed Jerry, throwing him onto the haystack. Everyone piled onto him, teasing him and roughing him up a bit. He sputtered and twisted but they held him until he said, “I give.” They then all had a big laugh, including Jerry.

Supper was on the table and everyone was seated in his or her special place. Abby looked at them and said, “All right, out with it! What’s going on?”

Everyone began talking at once, pointing to Jerry. Abby clapped her hands as she always did to get their attention. "Now, one at a time. Carl, you go first."

"Oh, let Jerry go first. I think I had to go first last time."

"All right Jerry lets have it! What's taking place?"

All the boys were busily eating, their eyes on their plates. Jacob looked wonderingly from one face to the next. He didn't have a clue.

"Well?" Abby questioned, looking at Jerry.

"I guess…well I just told the boys I'm gettin' married."

"What? What did you say?"

"I'm marryin' Carley White on May tenth," Jerry said, looking ill at ease. He didn't know exactly what to expect of his parents.

Abby looked at Jacob. He shrugged. He didn't know a thing. Jacob said, "Jerry, that's the best news I've ever had. I was beginning to think I was gonna have ta rent grandchildren if I was ever ta have any."

Everyone was patting Jerry on the shoulder and wishing him well. "Let's have a party Saturday all day and all night."

“Ya better talk ta Carley and her folks before ya go plannin’ parties. They may not have enough time off to attend a party,” Abby warned.

Everything was set the party was on. Everyone in the County was invited.

You could hear the fiddles, banjos, guitars and the harp being tuned up from a quarter mile away.

Carley was a pretty, buxomed girl of eighteen. Clear blue eyes and the whitest teeth you could ever expect to see. She was one of eight children of Hank and Sarah Furche. The Furche family was well thought of and lived good lives on their farm some eight miles from the Winter place. Everyone knew everyone for miles around and they were all there and ready to dance all day and all night.

The house was sufficiently large enough for all to find a spot to play, dance or gossip, which the ladies did. A whole hog and half of a steer cooked slowly all day on a huge out door spit. Part of each was highly seasoned and part was just salt and peppered. Home made seasoned tomato paste had been prepared to brush over the meat hanging on the spit and large bowls of it were placed on the table to dip the meat into. The table was laden with brown beans, cottage cheese, cakes and pies, cookies, plenty of fresh cold milk and pots and pots of coffee.

The music was going full blast. People were dancing and having a great time in general. Babies were crying and younguns were chasing each other and squealing. No one paid any attention to them except to change baby linens and to feed all from time to time.

The dancers formed a large circle. Jerry and Carley were shoved into the middle of the circle. One of the guests started the Circle Dance call. Everyone danced first to the right and then to the left. Jerry and Carley danced together within the closed circle. It was great fun.

A few of the older men went to the barn and took a couple of snorts of a brew Mr. Winter made of fermented apples or grapes. No one had more than one or two drinks. They were there to celebrate a coming wedding, not to get tipsy.

Monday morning found everyone back on track. They were still discussing the party and Jerry's coming marriage.

Jerry had rented a small farm, three miles east of his parent's home and was furnishing it piece by piece. Abby had given him and Carley many pieces of good furniture that had been stored in the attic. Carley's folks gave them the kitchen stove they had replaced as their family had grown. Friends and family were having quilting bees and were putting out a quilt a day.

Pillows had been filled with goose feathers and bed ticks filled with feathers for a feather bed had been finished and were ready for use. Dishes and pots were brought to Jerry's farm, along with blankets and muslin sheets.

They weren't going to need to buy a thing to get started. Of course, there would be many things they would have to get as they went along. Carley's mother had brought over two, room sized braided rugs, for their parlor and their bedroom. Someone had hung curtains at all of the windows.

Carley had never even seen the house but Jerry felt he knew her well enough to know what she liked.

Abby sent a letter off to Jenny telling her of Jeremy's coming marriage and all about the party. She also told her how the house Jerry had rented was being furnished and how cute it was.

"If only you could be here for the wedding, it would be perfect," she wrote. "I think Carl is getting serious about the Meeker girl. He has been going over there a lot. I'm hoping for a grandbaby within a year from now. Wouldn't that be wonderful?

How are you liking London? Do you intend to come back home after you finish your schooling of design? We all miss you so much.

Raye has been making noises about becoming a teacher. She never mentions any particular fellow. However she did say once that it was a shame you couldn't have cared for a nice young man like the Haskin boy. Maybe she has feelings for Patrick but is afraid you might feel bad if she kept company with him.

Patrick comes over a couple or three times a month to visit the boys but I've noticed him looking at Raye, when he thinks no one is noticing.

Have you met any interesting men over there or do you still think you may never get married? That would be a lonely way to live, I would think.

I hope you are happy and doing well in your studies. Please know we all love and miss you. Mama"

Jenny got the letter from her mother March second and thought, "I could make it home by Jerry's wedding day. If I did I would lose three and a half months of experiencing design and cutting. Oh I can't go back! I'll just have to write and explain to them how it is right now."

"Dear Family, I am so happy for Jerry and Carley. I do so wish I could leave right now. But I am at a very important place in my work that I would have to make up later. I just can't see my way clear to leave. I am receiving pay now for my own creations and have built up a small following.

Raye I am so glad you are thinking about becoming a teacher and I hope you find a nice fellow to like. You know Patrick Haskins often spoke of you, saying you were a very pretty girl and he liked the way you spoke right up when asked for your opinion. If you really got to know him you might find him to your liking.

I miss all of you so very much. I don't have time to even think about looking for a man. To tell the truth, right now, I'm just not that interested in marriage or a serious relationship.

I'm becoming more accustomed to London weather but I could sure use some of that good Kansas sunshine.

I haven't seen any Knights on white horses yet but I have visited a couple of castles. I've changed my mind about wanting to live in one. Although they are beautiful and opulent, they seem not to have warmth. They have so many rooms in them. Each room is large enough to swallow our house. There is just no feeling of friendly, cozy, normal living.

The people I have been privileged to know are all very nice. Their lifestyles are different than anything I have ever seen but they all treat me well.

I've got to go now. I've just sent off a large crate of things for each of you. I hope you all enjoy them.

I wish for lots of happiness to all of you and lots of grandchildren for Mama and Daddy.

Soon I may have some of my designs in some of the magazines you receive each month. Keep watch!

My best Love, Jenny"

****

CHAPTER 5

James Arlton was still peeved that Jenny had refused his company but had been out with Paul many times. He had seen them on several occasions dining. Each seemed to enjoy the other's company greatly. He had never approached her after she had rejected him at his home.

Why could he not get this girl out of his mind? It made him angry that he constantly thought of her. She was just a little Country Bumpkin, nothing he would ever consider for a relationship. So why was his mind cluttered up with memories of her fair skin, silky hair and beautiful eyes, full red lips and the way she walked? Damn!!

Jenny had her hands full of drawings and materials rushing to the cutting room. She hadn't seen anyone until she bumped smack into James Arlton just inside the doorway.

"Oh I'm sorry Sir," she said. "I should have paid more attention to where I was going," she bent down to retrieve her sketches and materials.

"Yes, you should have," James said, as he knelt beside her to help get her things in order again.

Jenny looked up to see James Arlton. "Oh, I didn't realize it was you Mr. Arlton. Again I'm sorry."

"I thought I told you, my name is James, not Mr. Arlton."

"I'm very late. Could we discuss this a little later?" she asked.

"Certainly!" he said, "Perhaps over dinner?"

"I'm, I'm not sure when I'll be finished. It will probably be midnight before I get out of here," she said on the run.

"Can we make it tomorrow around six p.m.?" he called after her. But she was already gone into the cutting room so he left his card and wrote on the back of it, "May I pick you up around six p.m. tomorrow?"

He gave the card to a young man instructing him to deliver it to Jenny in person. He gave the boy some coins for his services probably more than he made for a whole days labor.

Jenny, was so worn out when she finally finished at about eleven thirty, her back ached. Her eyes burned and her fingers were full of needle pricks as well.

The boy had delivered Arlton's card with the message to her earlier. She did not know what to do. She really did not wish to see

James. However he was Peggy Arlton's son and…well! "Oh darn," she thought, "I'll have to go."

James was right on time. He gave her a small nosegay of white rosebuds, tied with a pink ribbon.

"Where are we going?" Jenny inquired.

"Oh I thought you might enjoy watching the skaters on Pong Lake. I have a nice picnic basket packed up with an equally nice bottle of wine."

"Wine indeed," thought Jenny. "I'll be having no wine when I'm with you Mr. Arlton."

It was a nice brisk drive and the light from dozens of candles in glass globes, made the frozen pond glitter prettily. The food was delicious but most of it was foreign to Jenny. James offered Jenny wine in a crystal glass. She took it but barely sipped it.

After they had finished their food his driver loaded the empty basket. James then ordered the driver to a small theater. There they watched a comedy made up of three fat characters, two young lads and two spotted dogs. They laughed and thoroughly enjoyed themselves.

Jenny was very surprised to be so relaxed and happy. They talked about every thing, work, polo, business and design. They talked of Jenny's family in America and Jenny's dreams for the future.

She stated, "I do not think I'll ever marry. I just want to be a great designer and I think I can be."

"Can't you have both?" James asked.

"Not and do it well. One or the other would suffer," claimed Jenny.

James didn't say any thing concerning her dreams. He told her he felt like a leaf in a windstorm flitting first on place and then another with little or no control.

"Why do you say that? You have every thing a man could need," she said.

He just looked at her and changed the subject. James left her at her hotel lobby. He had not tried to kiss her or even hold her hand. She was very surprised and relieved.

****

CHAPTER 6

Bob Winter had taken on the job of Marshall for the Kansas Territory. He had a need to help people and this was his way to compensate for his youthful follies.

His first job as Marshall was to track down a man who had killed his own brother, in a fight over a woman. Bob could not even imagine striking any one of his brothers in anger or for any reason.

He had posters he put up all over the territory where he rode tracking Jack Bivens. He had mailed out posters to the surrounding states. It was a crude drawing of Bivens, with his vital statistics and a notice of 'REWARD' WANTED FOR MURDER!!

As Bob rode he remembered the twenty mile hike he had trekked while on the run. He remembered how tired and sore his feet had been. He remembered Sam and wondered where he was. It had been almost three and a half years since he had seen him. A lot of things can happen to a man in that time. Bob hoped Sam had reunited with whatever family or friends he may have had.

Being a Marshall was a dangerous job. Too many men would love to get rid of every law enforcement officer they ran across. So far Bob had not had to use the gun he had practiced with until he had become very proficient. Fast was important but being able to hit what you aimed at was even more to be desired. He was good!

Bob stopped at ranches, saloons and town sheriffs, asking questions. "Have you seen this man? When? Where?" He followed up every clue. The weather was as much his enemy as were the lawbreakers.

He was benefiting from his experience on the road as a boy. Bob paced himself and his horse. He knew how to dress and what supplies to carry.

He had just missed Bivens in the last town. Bivens had caused a free for all and was thrown out of town. Bob was weary but he kept on. He figured Bivins was just as tired and cold as he was and so was his horse. He had been following a horse track with a split shoe. The snow now covered the track but he continued on in the same direction.

It was just before daylight that Bob saw a hobbled horse close to a camp where a lone man lay. He examined the left front hoof and saw that sure enough it was the horse he had followed. Now if it was Bivins he could soon be headed back home.

Silently he approached the sleeping man. Drawing his gun, he lightly touched it to the man's forehead. When the man turned over Bob could see it was Bivins.

"Howdy Jack," Bob said. Put yore hands behind ya, careful like. I'd hate ta have ta haul a dead man all the way back."

Bivins obliged and got to his knees. "That's far enough feller," Bob said as he put the big cuffs on his prisoner. He looped a rope around Bivins' belly and cinched it up.

"Now stand right there while I git yore bedroll for ya. It gets a mite chilly. Ya will need it fore we get home.

Bob couldn't get much sleep. He had to keep one eye open to make sure Bivins didn't get loose.

Bob's beard was about an inch long and he needed a bath and clean clothes. The next little town they came to, Bob took his prisoner to the town jail to hold him there until he could get cleaned up. He left Bivins extra trousers with the jailer for Bivins to change into if he cared to.

Bivins had not said a word since Bob had taken him into custody but he accepted his clean clothes and a pan of warm soapy water.

Bivins wasn't a bad looking man. He looked very presentable after bathing and shaving. He smelled good too.

When Bob came for him he held his hands out for the cuffs and was led to his horse. Bob helped him up on his horse where he sat totally relaxed.

Finally Bivins offered, "Ya can rest easy, I'm not goin' any place. I deserve ta hang."

Bob wasn't taking anything at face value but he believed Bivins. Killing your own brother would be more than a man could carry around inside him.

When Bob fixed meals for Bivins he un-cuffed his right hand so he could eat but cuffed the left hand to the left ankle. Neither spoke, both seemed to be in deep thought.

Bob was awakened during the night by whispering. It was coming from where Bivins was laying, next to the fire. He heard Bivins saying, “No!”

Bob eased his gun out and quietly threw his cover off. He stood unnoticed in the shadow of a tree. “Easy boys! Step into the light of the fire. I don’t want to blow yore heads off, but I will.”

“Damn!” One of the fellows said, as he lunged toward the place where Bob’s voice came from. Bob now stood behind the tree and he slammed his gun barrel across the unknown man’s head. He could hear scuffling sounds from Bivins and some other person. Bob grabbed one of the men by the back of his coat pulling him off the other man. It was Bivins Bob had hold of. Bivins had his cuffed hands around the intruder’s neck, keeping him from leaving.

“Jack, what are ya doin’? Who is this man?”

“I don’t have a clue. He was just tryin’ ta git me loose so we could take off. I told him no, I wasn’t goin’. He tried ta take off and help his friend over there so I collared him.”

Bob tied both intruders back to back and waited until daylight to get a good look at them. "Who are ya fellers? What are ya doin' tryin' ta interfere with a Marshall and his prisoner?"

"Aww, we jist didn't like seein' anyone git hauled off ta jail, so we was jist lettin' him loose," the smaller boy said.

"How old are ya boys?" Bob inquired.

The biggest boy said, "I'm fifteen and my friend is sixteen."

"How come ya are the biggest if he is the oldest?"

"Hell, I don't know. We jist growed that way," he said.

"Where ya from?" Bob wanted to know.

"Jist back there 'bout four miles," said the fifteen year old.

"Don't ya ever talk?" Bob asked the older boy.

"Nope, not much. Junior talks enuff fer a dozen men. I jist wait cuz I know he will tell ever' thin' he knows. He always does."

Bob smiled to himself. "Boys, I'm gond ta let ya go this time. Jist remember, if I ever hear of ya getting' into any kind of trouble agin, I'm comin' back fer ya and I'm puttin' ya in jail. Do ya understand what I'm sayin'?"

"Yessir! We won't ever git into trouble no more huh Sandy?" Junior promised.

"Yep, that's right!" Sandy agreed.

Bob was remembering his young years and hoped these boys would learn a lesson from this.

Bob and Bivins started off again. They were almost home. "I want ta thank ya fer helpin' with the boys back there. Ya mighta got away."

"I told ya, I ain't goin' no place 'cept with ya ta jail. I killed my brother. I deserve ta hang."

"Jack, could ya tell me jist what happened 'tween ya and yore brother?" Bob asked.

"There was a woman we both liked. We got into a ruckus. When I hit him he fell and hit his head on a rock. He died, but he lived a few minutes and tol' me he forgave me. I jist took off runnin' til ya found me. I'm glad ya found me. I would'a come back anyway, soons I had time ta think on it."

Bob turned Bivins over to the Sheriff and wrote out a report part of which said, "The prisoner came willingly with me. He had the opportunity to get away but did not. In my investigation, I found the death was an unfortunate accident between brothers who loved each other. They just got a little hot under the collar and it resulted in one's death."

The judge would be through town the next Monday to hear the case. Bob would testify and Jack Bivins would most likely go free, Bob surmised.

Abby, Bob's mother had worried every minute Bob had been gone. She grabbed him and squeezed him so hard he thought he heard himself crack. He was glad to be home until Monday when he had to take off again.

A gang of outlaws were stealing cattle and driving them into Oklahoma Territory. The Marshalls in Oklahoma and Arkansas were getting posses together to come at the rustlers from all sides. Bob would take six men with him sworn in as deputies. All in all there would be eighteen lawmen in pursuit of maybe twenty five outlaws.

Monday, Jack Bivins was brought to the saloon where court was held. Judge Lane looked at the papers in front of him and asked, "Is the prisoner in court?"

Bivins stood and said, “Yes sir, I am here.”

“What do you have to say for yourself Mr. Bivins?” the judge said.

“Nothing Sir. I killed my brother. I deserve ta hang.”

Bob stood and said, “Yore Honor. My name is Bob Winter. I am Marshall of Kansas Territory. I’m the one that brought Jack Bivins in. I believe ya have my written report in front of ya. I will testify as ta the accuracy of my statement. There was no murder. It was an accident.”

The Judge read the report, looking at Bob said, “How long have you known this man?”

“‘Bout, two weeks. That’s how long it took me ta bring him in.”

“You did not know him before? You were not friends?”

“We still ain’t friends. I jist know he is not guilty from the investigation I did on this case.”

“Judge Lane looked at Jack and said, “Not guilty! Release the prisoner.”

Jack looked in total dis-belief at Bob then back at the Judge. “Thank ya!” he said.

Tuesday before daylight, the lawmen saddled up and left town. They rode quietly until they were well outside of town.

The Marshalls had kept what they were doing a complete secret. Even the deputies that rode with Bob or the other two Marshalls did not know what their job was going to be. They had volunteered for whatever was required of them. The Marshalls had not wanted any word of their plan leaking out.

Bob led his men to the far most north east corner of the State. They had stopped and fastened the sacks they had made on each of the feet of their horses.

"Keep yore mounts quiet. Don't let them whinny or snort. Hold their noses loosely so they can't push air through and warn anyone who might be close. Keep a close watch and ear for animals that might be comin' this way. Wait for a flare from yore left and yore right. When it comes be ready to ride and watch where ya shoot. We are after men driving cattle that don't belong ta them. We have friends ta our right and ta our left that are goin' ta help us capture a gang of maybe twenty five rustlers. Don't shoot our friends."

They sat and waited maybe thirty minutes when suddenly Bob could feel the ground quiver from hundreds of cattle feet.

"Mount yore horses and be ready to knock every mother's son of them out of their saddles. Try not ta kill them but stop them even if it means some men might die."

Daylight was just breaking when the herd reached Bob and his men. Flares had been lit and extinguished so everyone knew where friends were located and which were targets.

The cattle began circling not knowing which way to go with firing on all sides of them. The posse had been told to, "Ignore the cattle it's the rustlers we want." The cattle would be rounded up later and the brands returned to where they belonged.

The posse accounted for twenty three men. They didn't know for sure if they had them all. Two had been killed. Several had bullet holes in their shoulders, arms, legs, and rear ends. The men had done a good job.

Only two of Bob's posse had been hit and both were just flesh wounds.

Bob and the other Marshalls were well pleased except that one of Oklahoma's posse men had been killed. Arkansas men fared well also. Just some bragging rights wounds, nothing life threatening.

Each Marshall had a list of brands from his State. They sat about cutting their brands out and heading home. The rustlers were turned over to Sheriffs from six areas. Bob and the others had done their jobs. Now it was up to the courts and lawmakers.

****

CHAPTER 7

Carl had given his brothers the news that he was getting married next Christmas and needed help finding a small farm with a good house. Everyone had put out the word, but so far none had been located. He told Abby and Jacob that he wasn't having much luck, or really no luck at finding anything.

Jacob said, "Why don't ya take the forty acres down by the creek and build a log house. There are plenty of trees for logs and the creek for animal watering. We would have to dig a well for drinking but that's no big thing with all of us working."

Carl talked to Pansy and got her go ahead. The project got under way.

They still had to keep up all their work on the farm since they all worked for a salary just like anyplace else.

Neighbors from all over came and helped everytime they got a free hour or so. The house went up rapidly, the well was stubborn. They had dug four places and found no water. On the fifth try they got down about fifteen feet and hit a water vein. They then drove the well casing further down to get past the surface water table.

Abby had written Jenny that Carl and Pansy Wade were being married Christmas. She hoped Jenny would be able to come. "After all, you have been gone almost four years. Please try to come.

Raye had been seeing Patrick Haskin for months now. Everyone had been expecting an announcement from them at anytime so weren't surprised when it came.

September sixth, Raye said, "Mama, Pat and I are engaged. We would like a double wedding with Carl and Pansy, if they are agreeable."

"Oh I am so happy for you. Yes I think that Carl and Pansy might be thrilled to have a double wedding."

"Pat already has a house and has been working his farm for four years so he is well established. It's also close to the school I teach at. I'm so happy Mama. For awhile I thought I might be an old maid," she laughed.

Everyone thought a double wedding was a great idea. They all liked Patrick and were happy Raye had chosen him for their brother in law.

Frank piped up and said, "Looks like I'm next. I've asked Margie Townsley to marry me and she said yes, but not until next Easter."

Abby sat down, covering her face with her hands. "Oh dear. I was so eager for one of you to get hitched and give me grandchildren. Now all of you are getting ready to leave home and what will I do?"

Everyone went to her and hugged her. They assured her they weren't leaving her, but were bringing her daughters and an extra son.

Jenny was preparing for the long trip back home. She remembered how ill she had been on the trip to London and hoped she would not be ill going back.

She had many crates of finished dresses and gowns of all kinds. They were made of materials America's ladies would be able to enjoy and look pretty in. They could be worn at parties and dances as well as weddings. She also had some gorgeous, velvet on silk ball gowns for those who could afford them. She intended to stay in America for six months to set up a small dress shop, just to introduce her designs.

If they were not accepted by enough of the ladies then she would return to London or maybe even Paris and open a shop there.

Jenny would have preferred to wait for another year to come back so she could have been better known for her designs. Her Mother had been so adamant about her coming home for the weddings she had decided to come now.

She had also wanted to get away from Paul and James for a while so she could decide whether she wanted either of them or not. She had always liked Paul. She liked being around him and his son Peter was darling. But she only felt friendship for Paul.

James was different. He was like quick silver. She never knew what it was that he was after. He never spoke of love or commitment. He never asked her not to see Paul or anyone else. However, he looked like the black rain clouds back in Kansas, when she accepted invitations from others. It didn't matter if the invitation came from Paul or any of the few other men she occasionally saw. They were mostly buyers sent to look over stock and hopefully order vast amounts of garments for retail.

Paul's kisses were soft, sweet and un-demanding. James on the other hand, could be harsh and very demanding. His kisses were filled with a passion that caused Jenny to want to go further than they did, but she restrained herself.

Jenny had not yet told Paul, nor James that she was leaving on November sixth for America and would be staying six months or more.

She would tell Paul tonight and James Friday night when they went to the theater. She dreaded telling James. She didn't know what he might say or do.

Paul was devastated. "Oh Jenny, what will I do? I've become so accustomed to our dates. I just won't know how to cope for so long."

"I'm sure you will manage nicely," Jenny told him. "Anyway, you need to get out more, socially. You just let me take up all your time. Find Peter a new Mommy, start trusting again. You are a great person and you deserve the best."

James sat up very straight upon receiving the news and the muscle in his cheek contracted and he appeared to grind his teeth. "All right go. Stay as long as you wish. Do whatever it is that makes you happy. Wreck the start you have here. Let everyone forget you and your designs, be stupid." James climbed out of the carriage and held out his hand to her. He bent over her hand and kissed it lightly. He got back inside the carriage and ordered the driver to drive away.

Jenny had sent her crates ahead some three weeks ago. All she had with her in the way of luggage was one steamer trunk and a hand held carry all. It contained changes of nightclothes, lacy under garments, handkerchiefs, and toiletries. Her trunk would be put in her stateroom.

She looked around and saw Paul waving to her. James was nowhere to be seen. "Oh well," she thought, "At least now I don't have to make daily decisions as whether to see him or not. That should take a lot of pressure off my mind."

When she had gone to her cabin on the ship there were flowers everywhere, all signed, "Don't forget me." She couldn't even guess which had sent the flowers. It didn't really matter. They were beautiful and she enjoyed them.

So far on the third day out, she had not been seasick. Maybe she would be a good sailor this time. The long trip back to America was uneventful. Jenny was only ill a couple of times and she thought that may have been from the food. She had always had a finicky stomach.

The long trip from the ships docking was much more tiring and uncomfortable than the ship had been.

She arrived at her parent's home on December nineteenth. There was great happiness. Hugs, kisses and questions flew from every direction from everyone.

"Jenny, Jenny, my little girl. We are so happy to have you home again. My how you have changed!" Abby said, "And just look at your clothes."

Jacob held out his arms to Jenny. She flew into them crying, "Daddy, Daddy. I've missed you so much. I've measured every man I've met to you and they all come up short!"

Each brother took their turn hugging their sister telling her how glad they were that she was back.

The wedding preparations were ever ongoing, almost twenty four hours a day. The excitement was evident everywhere you turned.

Bride's gowns were being made with Jenny overseeing each step. A big reception was planned with all kinds of delicious foods. Special care was arranged for the children. A separate table was being set up for them in a different room.

There were to be thirty guests besides the family members on the three sides. All together, fifty grown ups and seventeen children, ages twelve and under had been invited.

The Winter home was large. The parlor was twenty foot by eighteen foot with the dining room adjacent to it about the same size. The den, where the men went to talk, smoke and get away from the womenfolk and the children had plenty of room with seating for about fifteen or so. The kitchen with its long table where the Winter family always ate their first meal of the day was sixteen foot by eighteen foot so there would be comfort afforded everyone.

Neighbors had brought in extra chairs, dishes, tablecloths and a couple of dozen pies and cakes. They should have leftovers for a week. The parlor and dining room were decorated with Christmas silver and red paper bells. The bells unfolded into wonderful looking wedding bells. Chains of paper were draped around the ceiling and had small tufts of cotton between each chain link. Every other cotton ball was colored red or silver. Long chains of popcorn balls were hung from the ceilings to be eaten by the children after the wedding. Holly with its bright red berries was everywhere and cedar boughs added color and the sweet smell of the outdoors.

The Brides were kept separate from the men which was no easy feat. The grooms were tended by their fathers and brothers and the brides were surrounded by giggling girls and women. The brides were very nervous but not nearly so as the grooms.

Finally, all were in their places. Abby played the organ. All eyes were on the brides as they entered through the door between the master bedroom and the dining room. A gasp went out when they saw the gowns Jenny had designed. They were the latest thing right out of Paris fashion books. Nothing like them had ever been seen in America.

They were made of beautiful shining white gossamer overlay with silk fitted gowns, hugging the bodies showing off the girl's youthful beauty.

Carl's and Patrick's eyes were shining with love for their beautiful brides. They had never seen anyone or anything so breathtaking as their ladies in those beautiful gowns.

The preacher was beginning his wedding prayer and listing the vows each said to their beloved. The brides were looking lovingly into their grooms eyes thinking how handsome they were and how wonderful their life would be.

The grooms were thinking of how they longed to have their wives alone, in their own home, away from every other living soul.

The people ate and they danced. The grooms were holding their new wives very close. Everyone talked at once. Jenny couldn't understand very much of what was being said, but everyone looked happy.

The brides and grooms left around ten p.m. Each couple was followed by family members, as well as friends. All were making so much noise but no one cared that they couldn't hear themselves think.

The party continued. Music filled the house and dancing feet wore the stain off Abby's wooden floor but she didn't care. She danced as much as most and more than some. When the musicians rested everyone gathered round and sang Christmas songs, giving praise to the Lord over all of them.

January fifth, Jenny set about trying to find out if the New York branch of Arlton's could give her some idea of what the public would bear. How receptive could she expect the American stores to be to stocking her merchandise which would be shipped from England?

Jenny had left her small dress making business in the care of two very capable ladies. Paul was keeping tabs on the business end as he had been doing for her over the last year.

She hated the train ride she must make to get to New York but there was no other way. The train rattled and jerked along making resting or sleeping next to impossible and it took forever to get there.

When they finally arrived at the train depot at New York City, she was told that much of her crated inventory had not caught up to her yet. They advised her that it would surely arrive on the next train, on the next day.

Jenny had been to so many House's of Design they were all jumbled up in her head. Only one had shown any interest at all and Jenny didn't feel as though there was much hope for her gowns in that one. Everyone was stuck in the past with their clothing style afraid of change. Jenny uncrated a dozen gowns and pressed them neatly. She had decided her designs had to be seen, felt and worn for perspective buyers. They simply could not envision their beauty by viewing drawings. After hiring a delivery concern for the entire day, with a clothes rack for her gowns and for several cotton dresses she set out. The deliveryman who drove the covered rig, also loaded and unloaded garments all day, but at the end of the day, Jenny had orders for a variety of clothing for every occasion. She left samples for people to order from of different fabrics and colors. Now she would wait. While she waited she sent off the orders for the things she had sold to her shop at home, along with a long letter to her employees and one to all instructing them to be ready to supply merchandise quickly.

"Paul, tell the girls to look around for cutters and seamstresses. They must be of the best at their craft and wholesome of character. I miss you and the girls. I miss my shop and my friends, but you most of all and I miss London, something I never expected to feel," Jenny confided to Paul.

A messenger arrived at Jenny's hotel on Wednesday with a note saying, "We would like to speak to you Miss Winter, concerning your American line. Could you meet with us at 2:00 p.m. tomorrow?" signed Ralph and Ralph Clothiers and their address.

Jenny danced around kissing the note and then holding it to her heart. "It's happening! It's happening!" she cried aloud.

Arlton's New York branch guided her through the maze of what felt like a nightmare of reparations; getting dress factories here in America to make ready-to-wear dresses and be ready to acquire the materials for the merchandise. She sent another letter to her home shop and had them start sewing cotton fabric dresses at once but not to turn away the tailor-made gowns for their London ladies. These we must keep happy at all costs.

There was a knock at her door. When she opened it James Arlton stood there with a small bouquet of violets, holding them out to her. "Could we go out to the lobby for a short chat?" he asked. Jenny didn't say a word but stepped through the door into the hall and walked ahead of James. She turned and looked at James inquiringly. "My, this is a surprise," she said.

"Yes, to me as well. I had no idea you were here until I went to the office and was informed that the wonderful Ms. Winter was making quite a stir in the garment industry here in New York. Can we talk over dinner this evening?" he asked.

"Oh James, I 'm so buried in work I can't see an end to it."

"You do still eat, don't you?" he smiled chidingly.

"Yes, of course, it's…Oh, very well, I can use a little reprieve from all this craziness," she agreed. "Yes, I'll be ready. Pick me up at the door."

James couldn't understand why he had lied about just finding out that she was in New York. He had kept tabs on her every move since she had landed in America some months ago. He was afraid she was not going to return to London and it made him frantic. Why?

Jenny was a vision of loveliness when he picked her up at the hotel door. It was almost impossible to keep from taking her into his arms and kissing her breathless. "Get hold of your self," he said to himself. "She's just a shop girl, no one you would ever want to be seriously coupled with," but deep inside, he knew better. This was the one and only for him. He could not deny it a moment longer. He was afraid to tell her how he cared. She was always so distant, cool, in a hurry to get away from him.

Jenny seemed to be thinking of things other than James. Her frown made those lovely lines over one eye that he longed to kiss away made swallowing difficult and he coughed, holding a linen napkin to his mouth. "Excuse me, please," he said.

Jenny was far from calm underneath her cool exterior. Firstly, she was very busy but had not expected to be so shaken at seeing James again. She knew his reputation with the ladies and his station in life. She had kept a bar up between herself and James, knowing nothing could ever come from any friendship with him. "Oh, I wish I had refused dinner with James tonight. I need my wits about me when dealing with all these people I'm trying to interest with my designs," she said to herself.

James was saying something. "Oh James, I'm sorry. My mind was on tomorrow's business. What was it you said?"

James looked at her and sighed, "I was just wondering if I might, uh, accompany you tomorrow when you visit different company heads. You know Alton's carries a lot of weight. It can help you in getting your foot in the door."

"Thank you James, but I'm determined to do this by myself, the face-to-face encounters that is. Alton's has already been a big help to me on several levels."

"How about dinner again tomorrow?" he asked. She wanted to, but knew she should not. She was just getting further lost in a play with no ending.

"I can't, James. I'll probably just get a sandwich in my room or skip it altogether."

"Jenny, you can't do that. It will ruin your health. You need at least two good meals a day not snacking on a sandwich and coffee."

"Don't do it. Don't do it!" her head was telling her but her heart, or at least her body, was crying out, "Yes, yes, yes!"

"Very well, dinner at six," she agreed.

James' heart beat fast and his feet felt like he was flying. She didn't turn him down. He would see her tomorrow and he was taking her where they could dine and also dance. He had to get her into his arms some way, even in front of other people if that was all he could manage.

When she had told him she was going back to America he had thought he would die. He stayed drunk for two days snapping at everyone, sullen, not talking for weeks. Finally, his mother Peggy told him he needed a vacation. "Why not go to America?" she advised. James knew that his mother knew or at least suspected he was gone on Jenny. Peggy had been a poor girl who worked as a seamstress for his father before they had married. She had felt so inferior with his dad being titled but it didn't matter. He pursued her relentlessly and practically forcing her. They had led happy loving lives until his dad had died twelve years ago. His mother never looked at another man.

"Tonight, I'm going to tell her I love her," he planned. He was scared. What if she would never see him again?

They went to a great dinner club. The music was wonderful and the couples were dancing, having a good time. "Shall we?" James motioned toward the dance floor, holding out his hand to her.

"Umm I guess so, but my feet are tired from being on them all day," she said. However, as soon as he took her into his arms her feet felt fine. "Oh my," she worried. He was going to know how happy she felt. She wouldn't look into his eyes.

She hardly tasted the food. Her mind was on trying not to show how she felt. Between dances she tried to talk shop but he wasn't having any of that. He told her how he had missed her and how much he had hated to see her leave London on that ship, where he had watched from behind a stack of freight and how he stayed drunk for two days and mean for weeks.

He told her the history of father and mother's marriage and life together and finally, how much he loved her and wanted her to marry him. Jenny sat very still and tried to figure out if she had heard right. Finally she asked, "What did you say?"

He came around the table to her side and he repeated what he had said guiding her onto the dance floor. Holding her as close as the public would approve of, "I love you, I love you, I love you. Marry me! I followed you here. I know every little thing that has happened since you landed in New York. I can't live without you. Answer me!" he demanded.

"Yes!" was all she could say. James picked her up and swung her around, laughing and shouting, "She said Yes, everybody! She said Yes."

Two weeks later Jenny and James left for London all business taken care of…happy as children at Christmas time.

****

CHAPTER 8

Weldon Winter was a six-foot, one-hundred-eighty pound fun-loving specimen of manhood and he loved the ladies, never settling on just one as his brothers had. He had fooled around with several young ladies, never even implying a serious relationship. He made it plain that no one was special to him.

Abby tried to talk to Weld but he would just laugh and say, "Mama, someday, I'll settle on one but not for a long time. Right now marriage is not an option."

"Son, don't you go and get some girl in trouble and ruin your life as well as hers."

"Mama, you worry too much," Weldon would say. He was the best worker of the Winter Clan, whistled and sang as he worked never complaining about anything. One day he came in, sat at the table with the rest of the family, and announced, "I'm leaving here and going to California. I just feel my life is in another direction. If I don't like it, I'll come back."

No one said a word for a full minute. Then, Jacob asked, "When did you decide this, Son?"

"Oh I've been thinking of it for a couple of years. I just had to wait until I was old enough to strike out," he stated.

"What do you intend to do in California? It really isn't very civilized out there."

"Yeah, I know. That's the biggest reason I'm going. There are no more hills to climb hereabouts. I've always craved excitement. I believe I'll find it in California."

Abby wiped her hands on her apron. "Is there any other reason you want to leave at this time?" she wanted to know. Weld knew what she was asking and he assured her.

"No, no reason at all, Mama." She looked relieved.

Weld intended to ride his horse until cold weather set in then take the train where it ran and whatever other transportation that was available. He had a warm bedroll, a frying pan, some fat back to fry the grease out of for trail food, jerky and biscuits his mother had insisted he take. He wasn't a coffee man so he didn't take anything to make it in. But he remembered Bob telling about how he and Sam had needed a pot, so he took a two-quart pot also.

He crossed into Oklahoma Territory the third day. He hadn't stopped anyplace at night, except to rest his horse and let him graze and catch a little sleep himself. He didn't push his mount just let his horse set his own gait.

Weld referred to his map often. He didn't want to stray too far from his mapped-out journey.

On the tenth day, he rode upon a camp of young riders. He asked them if he could sit a spell.

They all nodded. "Where are you going?" they asked him, to which he answered, "California". "You have a far piece to go," offered the eldest looking young man.

"Yep, but I'm just enjoying taking in the country. I've never been out of my home state of Kansas before. Where are you boys from?" he queried.

"Here and there," the oldest boy said.

"Going anyplace special?" Weld asked. "Nope, jist living off the land. Learning about being on our own."

"Don't you have families?" Weld questioned.

"Yeah, but we've all bad luck of one kind or another and decided to join up. We're all good with the cattle and pretty fair with a gun. It's just hard to convince the ranchers that we can do the job being so young and all."

"Ever think of joining the Army? They tell me it's a good place for a young man to start."

"Yeah, I did," said Danny, the older boy who did all the talking thus far.

"Maybe you should look into that," Weld offered.

Weld's horse was hobbled and was grazing close by. He didn't worry much about anyone taking off with him because he's a one-man horse and no one else could stay on him for long.

Weld was soon asleep with his head on his saddle his grub stuff at his side. When he got up the next morning all he had left of his pack was what had been in saddlebags where he had laid his head. His horse was un-hobbled and was grazing a way off. Weld whistled and Spike came trotting over to him. It was evident that the boys had tried to steal Spike without getting thrown or kicked. Anyway, he wasn't gone and Weld thought of Bob's feet when his horse had run off. They didn't take the pot but they got everything else. "What the hell!" Weld laughed, "I'll just use the pot instead of the frying pan." He shot a rabbit and cooked it over an open fire on a stick. It tasted great.

He whistled as he rode on through Oklahoma into the forest and on toward California. It was getting cold and soon he would have to start thinking about getting a ride on the train. He could bunk where his horse could be hauled if there weren't a lot of other horses in with Spike.

When he got to the railroad he inquired about where the train went and how much for him and his horse to California.

"What part of California?" the engineer asked.

"Oh, just anyplace where it's not too crowded and a man might find a job on a farm or something."

"Well, that could be almost anyplace in Californey young feller, but you orter stay away from the border with Mexico cause there's a heap of trouble around there most of the dang time."

Weld paid the fare and climbed aboard Spike. They were the only passengers in the boxcar. Weld fed Spike out of the feedbag furnished by the engineer.

When he crossed the great Cimarron River Weld felt a tinge of homesickness. He was almost out of Oklahoma Territory and well on his way to California. A great sadness overtook him. He wondered if he would ever see any of his family again. It seemed he had been in that boxcar for weeks before they stopped for water out in the middle of nowhere. In fact, it had been only one day and night. His head ached from the thick gray smoke that rolled into the door of the boxcar the jerking of the train and the sound of the clickety-clack of the train wheels.

Finally the train stopped and unloaded people and freight near San Francisco. There were people and horse drawn carriages and a few horseless buggies waiting picking up passengers or freight. No way was Weld getting off there; too many people, too much noise, too busy. "Nope, this is not for me!" he thought.

Two more cowpokes and their horses were loaded on to the boxcar along with Weld and Spike the horses on one end, snubbed up to the back wall. The two cowboys shared Weld's end of the boxcar. At least he had someone to talk to.

"Where you boys headed to?" Weld asked.

"Back home," one of them said. "We just drove a herd from the Bar-X-Z to be shipped on to Oregon."

"You'll be glad to get back home," Weld stated.

"Yep, it's been a long tiresome drive. Sleepin' in a real bed will shore feel real good. A couple of our boys quit as soon as we finished the drive. Now we are goin' to be short of help for awhile," the red headed man said.

"Do ya suppose I might be able to get on if I come with ya?" Weld asked. "Do ya have any experience with ranchin'?"

"Can ya handle a rope?" Jake asked.

"I was born and raised on a big farm in Kansas. I can do anything having to do with animals. I ride purty good and rope, brand and break horses…"

"Come along, giver a try!" the redhead, Jake said.

The other feller produced a deck of cards and they all kept busy entertaining themselves.

After the trio left the train at the junction they still had a ten-mile ride. Weld saw the grass waving in the wind and thought how Kansans would love to have grass like this at this time of year. Right now all the farmers would be feeding stock with no graze available until spring. He could see for miles. There were forests to the south, pasture to the right and left of them as they rode, lakes of sparkling water just ahead. They were now seeing cattle and horses that looked to be in the hundreds, if not thousands, all bearing the "Bar-X-Z" brand. All cattle were white faced with curly dark red bodies except for most of them having white stockinged legs halfway down from the knee. "Beef cattle, and healthy looking," Weld thought.

The ranch house was a huge two-story concern. It sprawled out into a 45-degree angle. It looked to be about six bedrooms from where Weld was looking. Everything was well kept and laid out with a breezeway between the kitchen and the main part of the house so as not to heat up the living area and the sleeping areas in the summer.

The two employees of the Bar-X-Z went directly to the main house to report how the trip went and how many they had ended up with at the stockyard outside San Francisco. The tally papers were checked and every thing came out even. Jake and Slade were good boys. Harve always knew that he could count on them to see everything was done as he ordered.

"Boss a feller rode along with us, hoping to get hired on. Seeing that we are two men short since Mark and Tim quit we just brung him along. When or if, you want to talk to him I can send him up."

"Now's as good a time as any bring him in," Harve ordered.

Weld took an instant like to Harve. He made him think of his father, clear eyes, square jaw, reddish hair.

"Were do ya come from, Will?" Harve asked.

"Just north of the Oklahoma border with Kansas. I was raised on a farm. I'm next to the youngest of seven boys. There's also five girls. My father salaried all of us boys from the time we reached sixteen and we had to give a full day's work for a full day's pay," Weld explained. "I'm a real good hand with animals and I'm good with a rope. I'm reasonably handy with a gun but I've never drawn my gun in anger. Being raised in a household of boys, I learned to hold my own in a donnybrook. I'm not lookin' for a career job as a cowhand. I'm intendin' to see as much life as possible but I'll give you my word that I'll never just quit without giving ya a month to hire a new hand."

"Sounds fair to me. Thirty dollars and found a month."

Weld stuck out his hand and shook Harve's hand. "The boys will tell you were to bunk and when to start in the morning. Breakfast is off the back room in the kitchen everyday, except Sunday. We don't work Sundays around here," Harve explained.

All hands went to the west fence line and worked steadily all day, stretching wire and putting in new posts when needed. Weld was a little sore. He hadn't put in a day's work since he'd left home some four months ago. He liked all the boys and sang and whistled as he worked.

"How many acres does this ranch cover?" Weld wanted to know.

"Oh, about a thousand, I think I heard Harve say," Jake offered.

"Whew!" whistled Weld, "and I thought our four hundred acres was a lot, but only about half of ours is under cultivation. The other two hundred or so acres hold beef cattle and horses. The cultivated acreage was lots more work." They raised wheat, oats, maize, cane and large gardens for canning-up. Fruit trees lined the lane instead of being an orchard shape. They raised around a hundred hogs for sale each year and sold three hundred eggs a day off six hundred hens or maybe five hundred hens and a hundred roosters. All the chickens were Rhode Island Reds. They kept geese and turkeys for meat and for feathers from the geese. Their preserved food was all kept in separate buildings where light didn't hit it except when foodstuffs were taken out or put in.

Abby always warned everyone to "keep the door closed on that building. Light causes spoilage," she warned. The smokehouse and cellar were always filled to capacity and the well house kept whatever needed to be kept cool that the cellar couldn't hold. With all those boys eating like ravenous wolves it took a lot of food twice a day, with snacks thrown in.

Harve got good reports on Weld. "He's a good hand. He never complains or sluffs off. Always seems happy," he was told.

Harve got to riding along side of Weld, talking to him about his family and how they worked their farm. He got some pointers that he thought he might try on the ranch. He really liked this young man. Harve's daughter had always been off-limits to any of the hands, Harve never allowing her to be present when they were in the house. As a matter of fact, his soon-to-be eighteen-year-old daughter had never had a caller. Even at the harvest or Christmas dances she was always made to sit by her mother, Gladys and only permitted to dance with men chosen by Harve which was so embarrassing to Gilly.

Harve invited Weld into the parlor to talk over ranch business. Gilly got up to leave, but Harve called her back. "Come here, Gilly. There's someone I want you to meet."

She looked startled, but kept her poise. "Yes, Father?" she queried.

"Weld, I'd like to present my daughter, Gilly. Daughter, this is Weld Winter. He works for us."

Gilly looked up at Weld and held out her hand. Weld touched his lips to her small hand murmering, "I am so pleased to meet you, Miss Gilly."

"Likewise, Mr. Winter," she dimpled up at him.

"Whoa!" Weld cautioned himself. "This is prime stock. No dilly-dallying here."

After that when Harve talked with Weld, Gilly was always sewing something or knitting sitting beside the fireplace glancing up to catch Weld's eye, from time to time. Gilly's secret dream was to leave the ranch and travel but she didn't dare let her father know how she felt, how she longed to go abroad and study music…real music, not fiddles and French harps. Gilly's mother knew of her dreams but gave her little hope of getting Harve to let her go to Paris or anyplace else. Gilly was her only child and both of her parents were so overly protective she could hardly breathe. That was why she nearly fainted when Papa had asked her to stay and meet Mr. Winter. Weld didn't appear to be a settling-down kind of man so if Papa was attempting matchmaking he had better read between the lines. Gilly bet herself that Weld had never had real feelings for any girl, and probably left a string of broken hearts behind him.

Gilly had never even been kissed unless you could count the Delong boy who sneaked a kiss on her neck while they were dancing.

Papa would have had a conniption, if he'd found out. She read a great deal, having nothing else to occupy her long days and nights. She read the great romantic novels and books on history, lots of books on music and art, biographies about the great painters, sculptors and composers.

Gilly knew that no hero was going to ride up and snatch her away to happiness and grandeur. She would just have to bide her time until her twenty first birthday. Then, she could go as she pleased and do as she wished and live off the money her Grandpa Pierce had left her. She wasn't really interested in marriage to anyone at the moment. But…

By roundup time, Weld had pretty well settled into the routine at the ranch and the long talks with Harve. He had also grown used to Gilly, saying "hello" and "Good evening" to her. He would always notice if she was wearing something new and would mention that she was looking nice in her pretty new dress or whatever. Gilly would accept his compliments but otherwise sat in silence while he and Harve talked.

Weld felt that Gilly didn't even notice when he left. He just wasn't used to being ignored by the ladies. Of course, he couldn't be his usual fun-loving self that he usually was around the ladies. Weld knew full well that if he showed any over attention to Harve's daughter he'd be off that ranch quicker than a cat could lick its behind, as the saying goes.

"Come up to the house about daybreak tomorrow," he told Weld. "We're going to town for supplies." Weld was there bright and early. The cook had packed a large basket, filled with food for them take along. They would spend the night at the hotel.

Weld was fitted up in his Sunday best. He looked strong and healthy and was whistling as usual, with a big smile on his face.

Harve and Gilly came through the door both dressed in city clothes. Weld had had no idea that Gilly would be going along and had been looking forward to a romp with the ladies around town. Well, he could still do that but he knew he would feel embarrassed if Gilly knew. However he really didn't understand his feelings. After all she hardly even knew he was alive.

Weld sat in the back of the wagon his feet dangling off the tail. When his legs would get tired he sat with his back against the side of the wagon, changing ever so often.

There wasn't much conversation between Weld, Harve or Gilly. She was trying to read a book but the wagon jostled so much it was difficult. Harve seemed to be pondering something deep.

Harve drove up to the Folder Grocery and Supply Store gave Weld a long list of supplies to give Mr. Folder to fill and told Weld he would get him a room for the night at the Royal Hotel. Weld saw him stop in front of the ladie's dress shop and let Gilly off, then drive on and stop again in front of a two story building on the right side of the street. He got out and entered through a side door. Weld couldn't see what the sign read from where he stood.

Weld handed the list to the man behind the counter and said, "Harve will pick them up tomorrow morning," and walked down toward the building that Harve had entered. It was some kind of building where four different businesses were listed. The one on the side door entrance read, "Dr. Hill, M.D."...Weld was alarmed wondering why Harve was going into a doctor's office. He didn't look sick and he didn't act sick.

"Well, I guess if it's anything serious he will sooner or later tell someone," thought Weld.

Weld went on up the street to the first saloon he came to. He stepped through the door and immediately stepped back. He had been told never to go into a saloon that was dark and or full of rough looking men. Too often men would be drugged and shanghaied and put on some ship, often never being seen again. Jake had told him of a good place, The Rustled Pony, to have an evening of fun, safely. The girls were pretty and the bar clean. When Weld waked in, he knew Jake was right. The long bar was made of a hard dark wood, polished and shining. Mirrors covered the entire wall behind the bar; glistening glasses filled shelves and whiskey bottles of a dozen different brands. Weld didn't know there were different kinds of whiskey. Mostly he had drank home-stilled whiskey and very little of that. He didn't really like the stuff and how it made some fellers mis-behave.

A pretty little redhead came up to Weld and asked, “Buy me a drink?”

Weld laughed and said, “Sure will, pretty thing,” and so the night began and lasted until bedtime, around midnight.

“Want to come up to my room for a goodnight snort?” the redhead asked.

“Why not?” he said with a twinge of guilt, as Gillie’s face flashed before him.

It had been a very long time since Weld had been with a woman and he stayed all night making happy love to a bar girl with red hair. He had not even gone to the Royal Hotel where Harve had said he would make him a reservation for a room.

Weld was in front of the store waiting for Harve and Gillie when they drove up. Harve still had that preoccupied look he had had allday before but he was his usual self, by the time they were on the road again.

“Where did ya go last night?” Harve asked. “I asked for ya a couple of times at the desk but was told ya hadn’t checked in.”

"Oh, I met some people and ended up stayin' the night with them," he said. Harve knew exactly what had happened but did not pursue it further.

Gilly sat very straight and said not a word all the way back to the ranch. She pretended to read her book and looked neither left nor right. The wagon was unloaded and Weld took it back to the barn and unharnessed the horses, watering and feeding them before he went to the bunkhouse. The boys were full of questions on how he made out what he did and who he did it with.

He told them he had gone to The Rustled Pony had a nice time with a redhead but he would not give any details. A man doesn't go around kissin' and tellin'!

Harve called Weld into the house. "Have a seat, Son," he said looking a little excited, Weld thought. "I ordered one of those new-fangled horseless carriages," Harve confided to Weld. "It's a birthday present for Gilly. We are havin' a big shindig Sunday next to celebrate and I want ya to come."

"Oh Harve, I don't think that would be appropriate. I'm just a cowhand like the rest of the boys and I'm afraid they'd feel left out. I sure don't want any hard feelings between us. We have to work together and get along in order to do you a good job."

"Weld, they are delivering the dang thing on Saturday and I was hopin' you'd allow the fellers' that's bringin' it to teach you how to drive it. I'm too danged old. I'd run it into the barn or fence or house."

"Harve, I've never even rode in one of those things. I don't know a thing about them," Weld informed him.

"I'll let the boys know I need ya to show Gilly how to handle the darned thing, and invite them to share in the vittles and give them a couple of bottles of brew each. It'll be all right."

"But, I'm tellin' ya, I don't know how to herd those things around," Weld stated.

"Oh, don't worry. By next Sunday you'll be an expert," Harve assured him.

Early Saturday morning two automobiles drove up to the barn on the ranch, as instructed. They were met by all the cowhands. They walked around and around the machine, touching it and laughing. "What do ya feed 'er?" they asked, laughing at their own wit.

Weld went up to the main house and informed Harve that someone wanted to speak with him. Harve put his hat on and left the house, walking rather quickly for him.

"How does she look?" he inquired of Weld.

"Well, it shines and it's a might noisy, and that's about all I can say…not ever having anything to compare it with."

"Howdy, fellers," Harve said, as he reached the barn. Weld was right. It was colorful, shiny black with bright yellow wheels. There was only room for two passengers at a time. That didn't seem very practical to Weld but he guessed it suited Harve. The men who delivered the machine brought Weld and Harve to the front of the machine and pointed out all the features of the black beauty. One of the men told Harve to sit on the passenger's side and he would show him how to drive it. "Nope," Harve said. "Show Weld. He'll show me later."

Weld shook his head in a helpless motion. "I'm tellin' you fellers, I know nothin' about this durned buggy. I've never even touched one of them until now."

"Oh, come on," one of the men said. "There ain't nothin' to it. I learned in a couple of hours. You turn this knob to start the motor and pull this lever to go forward. Step on that right pedal to stop and this to back. Put both hands on this wheel and turn it to the right just a little and to your left just a little. Keep to the right of whatever road you're on. There now, see how easy it is?"

"Nope, it don't look easy to me but change places with me and I'll try it," Weld said. When Weld was behind the steering wheel he tried every lever and pedal before he started the motor and headed down the long lane that led to the junction. At first he was way off the side to the right, then to the left.

Finally he thought, "It's just like riding a horse or driving a horse-drawn wagon. Pull a little one way and if it don't stay on the right side of the road pull a little to the left." Weld stopped and started several times, backed up and took off again. The lever made it go faster or slower. Weld felt pretty good by the time they got back to the barn but worried about driving where the carriages were motor or horse drawn.

Harve had the cowhands hitch up a wagon and a buckboard and four cowhands on horses to ride in both directions as Weldon continued to practice. He was getting the hang of guiding, starting and stopping.

Sunday afternoon the party was in full swing with music, dancing and eating. Everyone was wishing Gilly a happy birthday and was handing presents out to her.

"Gather around everybody and Gilly will open her presents," Harve ordered.

There was much oooing and ahhhing as she undid each package.

When Harve handed Gillie his present it felt so light Gilly could not imagine what it might be. Enclosed was a card which read, "Go outside and claim your present." Signed Mom and Dad.

Gillie ran to the door and threw it open. Weld was standing beside Black Beauty, holding one hand toward her and the other toward the car. It was 1908 and her first new motor carriage.

She looked toward Harve curiously and back toward Weld. "It's yours!" he said.

She walked slowly toward the automobile touching it with slender fingers as she circled and climbed up onto the seat. “I can’t drive this,” she said.

Weld offered, “I will teach ya, if ya will allow me!”

Gilly looked at her father and he nodded.

She noticed there was only room for two in the vehicle and wondered how Harve had ever decided to trust her alone with Weld.

She had made it a point not to be absent at the meetings between her father and Weld ever since his trip into town.

“When can I try it?” she asked.

“Now is as good a time as any, scoot over.” Weld climbed onto the driver’s side and began to show her all the knobs and levers. He showed her how to push the brake and how to work the reverse. “This lever makes it go faster or slower and it guides just like a horse. Pull a little to the right to stay on the right and gently to the left to keep her straight.” They had driven about a mile when he stopped and changed places with Gilly after turning back toward the house.

She was very nervous but ready to try the thing out. At first she pulled too hard and was all over the roadway and then stomped on both pedals killing the motor. Weld just spoke softly and got her back in control. By the time they stopped in front of the house, Gilly was driving with a little more confidence but she didn't want to try it alone and the thought of going into town scared her to death.

Everyone was excited and asking questions in a steady stream. "What does it feel like? Were you afraid? Did you get in the ditch? Etc. etc.

Gilly was very happy and thanked her parents several times. She wondered about Weld. He had not said anything except to explain the rule and motions it took to drive. She wondered if Harve had given him orders not to speak of any thing personal or maybe he just wasn't interested. Well if he thought she would ever make the first move he had better think again.

Weld had made a concerted effort to be very impersonal. He didn't want Harve to feel he had to guard Gilly from him. Gilly was a courageous young woman and beautiful, but Weld did not frolic with good girls and he was not interested in firm relationships. He had many places to go and much to do in his remaining life span.

****

CHAPTER 9

When Jenny and James arrived in London being met by Paul, Jenny hugged Paul and told him how much she had missed him. James and Paul shook hands and chatted about the trip over and about business problems at Jenny's shop. "Not really problems," Paul explained, "just overworked employees with so many orders piling up there seems to be no end in sight."

Jenny was in a hurry to get to the shop and decide what had to be done first.

"Oh Miss Jenny, it's so good to see you and just in time I might add," Sylvia said. "We have been able to interest Sheldon's factory to make and distribute our American line direct to jobbers in America at a rate you can live with. You however must visit them in person. Now that you are here you may be able to get an even better deal."

James had gone home to see the family and to break the news that he and Jenny intend to be married just as soon as Jenny can get her business affairs in order, probably in April.

"Well, it's about time," Peg said. "I thought you would never smarten up to the fact that you were in love with her. Jenny will make you a good wife. She has a mind of her own and you will never be able to take advantage of her just because she is your wife."

"I know that Jenny is of that special breed of career women just as you are mother. Maybe that's why I fell in love with her," James said.

"No, you fell in love with her because she wouldn't chase you and did in fact ignore you while others pursued you and gave in to you. I hear she is really doing wonderfully with her line of design."

"Yes she is. She worked feverishly in America setting things up on that end, now being able to fill the orders is the problem. She has a market for every garment she can produce."

"Maybe I can help," Peg offered, "until she can get her own going."

"Oh mother, that would be wonderful if you could and it would help to set the wedding date up too." James reasoned.

There were several letters from home waiting for Jenny. She didn't have the time to open them as of yet and she worried that something important might be happening in the family. Tonight she just must get to her personal mail as she had taken care of all the business mail. She kicked her shoes off as she went through her door.

One letter was from Raye and her husband. She had written just happy feelings and best wishes to her and James upcoming marriage.

She opened a letter from her mother. Abby was worried over Weld taking off months ago and she had only received one short note from him. It said he was on a ranch outside of San Francisco, California. He said he liked his boss and that he had learned to drive a horseless carriage. “My children are all going off to find lives of their own and you know Henry has gotten engaged as well. I’m so glad Mildred, Harriet and Rosie are small. I miss all my children very much when they are no longer living under my roof.”

There was a letter to her from Weld as well. “Hi Sis,” he began. “I’m having such a lot of fun here on the Bar XZ Ranch. My boss is a wise old man, not too old, forty seven I think but smart as they come. He has a thousand acres and utilizes every inch. His house ain’t as big as ours but it’s a lot richer looking. He and Gladys have only one child, a girl of about eighteen I think. I learned to drive one of those new fangled horseless carriages. On the way here from Kansas I got most of my cookin' stuff stole. They tried to steal Spike but ya know him. No one rides him but me. It looked like he mighta throwed someone and kicked about some. I brought him with me on the train after we got into the Oklahoma territory. That's where I met up with the fellers that work for Harve. I was thinkin' that someday I might go to England and see how you folks live. Write to me in care of Bar-X-Z, San Francisco, California.

Stay Happy,

Weld

A month had flown by so fast Jenny just didn't know where it had gone. Arlton's had made her job mush easier. She had time to shop around for the best deal she could get and not be pressured into something less than she needed or wanted.

Jenny hardly had a moment with James and he would some times grow impatient when she was loaded down with business. "It just cannot be helped," she explained to James. There just are not enough hours in a day to get everything attended to."

She was setting this coming Sunday aside to be with James all day but she had not been able to contact him yet to tell him so. She put the word out to Peg to tell James of her plans if she saw him.

Jenny wrote to her family and included Weld's letter to her. She also answered Raye's letter and gave her all the gossip on her end.

She wrote Weld that she would love to have him come to London but she didn't believe there were ranches here. At least not the kind he was used to but there were places that handled horses for the polo crowd. She was sure he could find some kind of work and "Weld, write mama more often and in more detail."

James had gotten Jenny's message and had made elaborate plans for dinner, dancing and an after hour's drink at a friends flat.

He was hoping to be able to hold her close and tell her how much he loved her and to convince her to move up the wedding date. Peg could make all the arrangements. Jenny would only have to design her gown and have it stitched up.

Jenny was ready and waiting at six p.m. when James called for her. She was dressed in a beautiful fitted gown of midnight blue. She seemed to glow in the candle- light, James thought.

They ate, they danced, they talked and they laughed.

James instructed the driver to drive to his friends place.

Jenny asked, "Where are we going? I must get some sleep. I have a full day tomorrow."

"Oh it's a secret," He said as they drew up in front of a stone building in a better part of London.

James helped Jenny out and guided her through the large double door. Once inside they moved toward a wide carpeted stairway. James led her to an open door on the right. Candles glowed softly on a bottle of wine and two glasses. He took her wrap and seated her kissing her hair and squeezing her shoulders briefly.

Jenny could hear music from someplace near playing softly. James held out his arms to her. "Shall we?" he asked.

She rose and walked into his arms being held tightly against his body for the first time. Jenny pushed against his chest trying to put a little distance between their bodies.

"It's alright," he assured her. "The door is open and after all we are engaged."

She relaxed a little but still kept at least a couple of inches between them.

"Jenny, Jenny!" James breathed. "I love you so much. I need you. I want you with every fiber of my being. Let me love you, please let me."

"I can't James. I was taught the only way to give ones self is on their wedding night. My mother would die if she ever thought one of her girls was going all the way before marriage."

"But baby, we will soon be married."

"Soon yes but not right now," she argued.

"Just kiss me really kiss me Jenny, just once, please."

"I have kissed you many times," she stated.

"But not deeply, letting yourself go," he complained.

Jenny really didn't understand what James meant. She had allowed him to kiss her lips and to hold her near. "All right, I'll kiss you but you will have to teach me how to let go as you said. I've never kissed any other than you except Paul in a friendship way."

James pulled her against his throbbing body kissing her eyelids, forehead, face and finally her lips. He started slowly, tenderly, gently, using his tongue to part her lips, which caused Jenny to pull back. He gathered her closer still kissing her deeply, passionately causing Jenny to have feelings she had never experienced before. She bowed her self into him and clung to him. He was breathing hard and was telling her how wonderful she felt to him so close to him, how he loved her. She heard the word now through a haze of passion and willed herself to twist away.

"No! Not now James. It is wrong James, wrong!"

"Nothing is wrong if we love each other my little darling," he said.

She beat against his chest with her small fists crying "No, no James. I won't, I can't. Stop it right now. I mean it! Stop!"

James released her standing back breathing hard a look of frustration on his face. "I'm sorry I just got carried away. It won't happen again. April is too far away. Peg said if you made the dress or designed it and had it put together she would arrange everything else. You don't have to do a thing, how about it?" he asked.

"Give me a little time to think. I'll get in touch with Peggy and talk over details, don't pressure me so. I've got so much going on right now I can't think straight. I must send invitations to my family and friends at home. I really don't expect them to make that long ship ride but I must allow time for them to get here if they want to. By the time I can send them an invitation and they could get a ship out it will be April any way," she explained.

James hung his head and looked like a hurt little boy that had just been told there would be no Christmas this year.

Jenny wanted to cuddle him and tell him everything would be all right but she didn't. She was afraid he would become aroused again and she was afraid she wouldn't be strong enough to make him stop.

"It will probably be safer if we don't go out much. When I touch you dancing or even in or out of your chair…Well, I just love you so much I cannot keep my hands off from you."

Jenny was offended. She thought, "All he cares about is my body, not me."

She spoke to Peggy about the wedding arrangements and about the situation with James.

"Men are different than we are my dear. We love with our minds as well as our hearts. Men love with their physical urges and their hearts secondly. It's the way they are made. They measure their manhood by their bedroom activities how well they perform and how females react to them. Try not to be offended. It isn't something they handle very well."

Jenny felt much better after her conversation with Peg. She had, had nothing and no one with which to compare James' actions with and had taken it personally. She still could not understand men and she really didn't understand her feelings when James held her so close and kissed her so thoroughly. She felt as though she wanted to push him down onto the floor and lay on top of him with no clothes on. She tingled all over. It scared her.

Jenny and James were never alone again. They shared dinners and sat in on business dealings. James was careful not to hold her too tightly or kiss her too deeply. Still he was suffering needing to have her wholly, not just tiny kisses and surrounded by dozens of people.

Jenny had received letters from back home. None of the family could come but sent presents and wishes for their happiness.

Weld was the only one who might show up. "But don't expect me till you see me at the door," he said.

There were just five more weeks till April fifth. Jenny was beginning to get nervous. James had so much experience and she had none. What if she didn't please him? She had no idea what was expected of her. "Oh dear, I should have had mama tell me what to do. It's too late now," she thought.

Her dress was almost finished. It was yards and yards of white silk with lace and ribbons with a long train of finest silk. Her veil was of Irish lace. She had already had a fitting and it fitted well and looked wonderful on her.

James bought a motor carriage and finally convinced Jenny to ride in it. He came to pick her up on Sunday, she almost changed her mind. She had been watching the machines on the streets of London. They just do not look safe and they go so fast no one is safe. The horses rear up and run uncontrollably and women and children run and scream.

James left downtown London driving toward his home. There were much fewer conveyances, either horse drawn or motor on his route.

Jenny was feeling very adventurous and agreed to try to drive around the grounds if James would stay beside her. That was in case she forgot to stop or go slower or something equally as drastic.

They were having great fun. Jenny would yank the steering wheel too hard then yank it back weaving all over the grounds of the castle. Finally she got the hang of steering but starting and stopping or going backward was still a problem.

"Oh Peg, it is so much fun and takes so little time to get here from my hotel."

"Peg smiled and said, "Yes it is fun and I save so much time driving mine."

"You have one of your own, really Peg? You really do?" Jenny asked. "Maybe I should learn to drive well and get one for myself. I seem to always be late everywhere I go."

"Well Jenny, what you need is to stop taking on more than you can handle in a day, everyday," Peg said.

"I had my last fitting of my wedding gown. It is so pretty."

The ballroom was already decorated and the many chairs were sitting in straight rows, ready for the many expected wedding guests.

The raised stage was shining like a gold piece. The dining room was set up for the reception. There were long lace covered tables with beautiful chairs lined on either side of each table. Wedding souvenirs were beside each plate and flowers were everywhere.

"Tomorrow is the day. Tomorrow I'll be Mrs. James Arlton, no longer Jenny Winter," she thought. "Can I be what James and the Arlton family expect me to be? Will I please James? Will I enjoy lovemaking? What if I don't?"

The driveway to the castle was framed by men in armor riding pure white horses. The doorman held a gold-headed staff about seven feet in height which he struck on the floor before announcing each guest.

James had told his mother Peg of Jenny's daydreams while a child on her father's farm. She waited for a knight in shining armor to come riding in on a white horse to rescue her and take her away to his castle.

As Jenny was driven toward the castle door she cried as she saw all the horsemen just as she had dreamed so often as a child. James had arranged all this. She had never told anyone else. A surge of love for James ran through her whole being.

The footman led her inside holding her train off the floor. Peg and the two bridesmaids hurried to her and began tugging at her gown and veil to get it just right. Everyone oood and ahhhhd at how pretty she looked and her gown was the most beautiful they had ever seen.

The music started and she took Paul's arm, he was giving her away in the absence of her father. Four small girls in pink silk ankle length dresses scattered rose petals as they walked behind Paul's five year old son who was carrying the rings on a silk pillow about eight inches square. Two bridesmaid and Peg walked right in front of Jenny and Paul wearing pink dresses the same as the flower girls.

"James is so handsome." Jenny thought as she walked in step with Paul. "Please let me be worthy of carrying the Arlton name and help me to be all that James needs me to be."

As James watched Jenny walk toward him he wanted to call to her to walk faster. He was so eager to make her his wife. It seemed to be taking forever for her to reach him.

Finally, she was standing beside him holding pink rosebuds tied with white ribbon streamers in her small hands. "She is so beautiful," he said to himself. He hardly heard what was being said. He was waiting for the, "You may kiss your bride" part.

Finally the preacher said, "I now pronounce you husband and wife. You may kiss your bride."

James lifted her veil turning it back over her head. Gently he folded her into his arms and slowly kissed her. "I love you," he whispered.

"I love you," Jenny told him.

There was quiet a stir with everyone talking at the same time, then the music started and James claimed Jenny for the first dance after her train had been disconnected. He wrapped both arms around her waist holding her so close she could hardly breathe. After their dance they went to their dressing room to change into different clothes so they could dance or sit at the table comfortably. It seemed to Jenny that at least fifty men had danced with her. To Jenny's disdain James was being mobbed by the ladies. She felt a stab of jealousy. After all, he was no longer fair game.

James claimed her for the last dance then guided her to their area of the castle. They had totally separate living quarters from the rest of the castle with private entrances.

No one would invade their quarters and the servants would come only when rang for.

Jenny was uneasy. She didn't know what she was supposed to do. There was a sheer nightdress lying across the huge bed with fur-trimmed slippers to match. She was afraid. James could see right through the nightdress.

James came back into the room seeing she had not undressed yet. He pulled her off the bed and slowly began undoing her many buttons letting her dress drop to the floor. "Step out," he said. She did and he began to unlace her corset then removed the many petticoats. She crossed her arms over her chest and blushed. He kissed her face, her lips and her shoulders and gave her a little push toward the dressing room handing her the nightdress. "Finish undressing in there." He said pointing toward the dressing room and put this on.

Jenny was so afraid and so embarrassed. She had never been disrobed in front of anyone before, male or female.

When she didn't come back to where James lay he called to her. She did not answer. He knocked on the door also getting no answer. He entered the dressing room finding her sitting on the vanity bench her back to James.

"Jenny, come to bed." She just sat there not moving or saying anything. He walked over to her picked her up and kissed her tenderly. "It's alright baby. I'll be very careful with you."

"But I don't know what to do James. I can tell you have done this a lot the way you removed my garments knowing where each piece opened."

"Yes I've been around some and I have undressed women but I have never loved any of them. I love you," he said.

He turned down the coverlet on the bed and told her to get in. He put all the candles out except one across the room putting them in shadows.

He turned toward her undoing the ribbons that kept the sheer nightdress closed and slipped it off her shoulders. He kissed her face, ears and lips and moved on down to her throat which made Jenny gasp. She was getting that feeling again. She wanted him to kiss her harder and to touch her. He seemed to read her mind and kissed her passionately. She was pulling his head back to her mouth when he tried to move it lower. She remembered thinking she should probably stop him.

"Jenny, I love you, I love you," and he waited for Jenny to say something.

"If I had known this was what lovemaking was about, I would have married you the first day you asked me," she said.

"My baby darling, I had a hell of a time not raping you. I just wanted you so badly, I haven't been able to sleep for months."

Jenny was rubbing her hands over his chest, kissing it and then his lips.

James had worried that Jenny might be frigid but no way was she. My darling beautiful wife is a woman among women. He was so lucky. He knew he would never stray. He had everything a man could ever want.

****

CHAPTER 10

Weld was appointed to go everywhere Gilly went in her motor carriage. He always kept the conversation impersonal. He pointed out small animals, flowers, another carriage anything so long as it wasn't about himself or Gilly. She seemed to try once in a while to talk about his sister in London getting married or Jenny's business holdings but Weld would just shrug his shoulders and change the subject.

"I would love to go to London or Paris or just any place away from this ranch." She told Weld. But Weld wouldn't be drawn into any discussion about going any place.

Harve would look at Weld as if he expected him to say something about Gilly, but Weld didn't.

Gilly told Harve all about everything they talked about and added, "Weld Winter is not the least interested in women."

Harve knew that wasn't a fact. All the boys talked of how the ladies chase after Weld and how he spends his time off with a number of ladies. It must just be because of his loyalty to his boss. There was no other reason he wouldn't like Gilly.

Harve wanted to get his daughter married and settled and he wanted to be around to make sure some feller wasn't just after her money. He knew Weld would make Gilly a fine husband and would take good care of the ranch. "Well…Time will tell," he thought.

Weld had been thinking on taking a trip to London to visit Jenny and look over parts of some other countries. He gave Harve a month's notice telling him he just needed to see more of the world. Maybe he would hate it and come back right away but maybe he would want to stay.

"I sure hate to have you go Weld. I've grown quite fond of you, sorta like you were the son I never had. If ya come back will ya come by and see us?"

"Sure will Harve. I've been happy here. I've made some nice friends and had some good times. Yep I'll come by," he promised.

"Have you mentioned to Gilly that ya are leavin'?"

"No but I'll make sure to say good bye before I take off."

Friday, before Weld's ship was due to leave on Monday, Gilly asked Weld to go to the mailbox with her.

"Sure thing," he said when they started off. "This will probley be my last time to go anyplace with ya."

"Why is that Weld?"

"I've told Harve that I'm leavin' Monday for London to visit my sister and to look over that part of the world. I've stayed too long in one spot, got too comfortable and had grown too fond of Harve. I only intended to be here a couple or three months and it's been over a year."

"I will miss our outings. Now I don't know who papa will allow me to be chaperoned by."

"Oh I think you drive well enough to go alone." Weld offered.

"Now you know very well papa wouldn't let me go anyplace by my self. Weld, would you leave your sister's address with us? I'm rather concerned about papa's health. He just doesn't seem quite right health wise, she stated.

"Of course!" Weld said. "Has he said anything about feelin' bad?"

"No, he never complains, but I just know something is wrong," she insisted.

Weld walked onto the deck of the London bound ship at nine a.m. looking forward to the adventure but more than a little worried about Harve.

He met a whole slew of both men and women on deck and struck up conversations with some of them. He wasn't getting sick but a lot of people were very sick. He remembered Jenny saying she was ill the whole trip the first time but the second time she fared well and was able to enjoy the sea breeze and the cool sunny days.

He had left Spike with Harve. He knew Spike would be cared for no matter how long he was gone.

Weld hadn't told Jenny he was coming. All he had was her business address and the name Arlton, but he knew he could find her soon enough.

****

CHAPTER 11

By the time the ship landed in London, Weld had tanned even more and looked healthy, (which he was) and excited. He got a map of London and found Arltons'. He hired a carriage and looked the area over as he rode to the school of designs.

The ladies eyed him when he entered wondering where the fine specimen of manhood was from and what did he want? He didn't look like a city feller so he wasn't a jobber.

Weld rang the bell at the counter and one of the women came in and ask, "May I help you?"

"I hope so. I'm looking for my sister Jenny Winter, er I mean Arlton. Can you tell me how to get to her house?"

"Yes, but that won't be necessary. Jenny is here in conference. She will be finished in about three minutes. I'll tell her she is wanted out here. Have a seat Mr. Winter," the woman offered.

Jenny came out of the conference room a slight frown on her face. Who could be needing her here? She looked around and spied Weld. She ran to him throwing her arms around his neck. "Oh Weld, why didn't you let us know you were coming? Come let's go home. I want you to meet James. He is wonderful. I know you will like each other."

She led him to her motor carriage and told him to get in. She expertly started and drove through the streets of London. There were many carriages on the street. More of which were motor vehicles than horse drawn conveyances. Weld felt perfectly safe with her driving. She drove well and didn't get flustered in the downtown traffic.

"Where do you live way out here?" he asked.

"Oh it's just a short distance more," she smiled.

When she turned into the gated drive he couldn't help but wonder where in this area of huge castles she could possibly live.

She drove to the entrance on the north side of a castle stopped and said, "Come on." He stepped out of the carriage and followed her into the doorway where on either side of a very wide hall were huge paintings that covered the walls. "Wait in here" she said as she ushered him into a room with two fireplaces, not lit as it was too warm. It was furnished with beautifully covered chairs and long soft cushioned sofas to sit on.

"Who lives here?' he questioned.

"Only my husband and I," she said.

"My goodness! What about the rest of this…this…?"

She smiled and said, "Castle?"

"Yes, castle. Why are you living here?" he demanded.

"Because it is James' family home. His father was royalty and James now bears his title since his father died."

"Royalty! What kind of royalty?" he almost shouted.

"My husband is Lord Arlton. I am his wife, Lady Arlton. But we only answer to James and Jenny."

"I am the brother to a royal someone? That just won't fly," he said. "Who is ever going to believe a story like that?"

"Just don't tell anyone." She advised. "We are just two very happily married people named James and Jenny."

Weld was whistling as he inspected Jenny's home. "How could anyone feel comfortable in this cavernous, cold stone dungeon?" he thought to himself.

The room he had been given was large enough for a family of four. What a waste.

James had returned from where ever he had been. Jenny told him she had a surprise for him.

"Ummm, I love surprises. I love you," he said as he kissed her and kissed her and kissed her until she was breathless. He picked her up and started for the bedroom.

"No! No, James. We have company. We can't," she squealed.

Weld stepped into the first room Jenny had taken him to. Seeing Jenny held in a good-looking man's arms he turned to go.

"Come in Weld. I want you to meet James."

Weld walked to where Jenny now stood beside the tall man. James walked toward Weld holding out his hand.

Weld gripped his hand firmly laughing. He said, "This is beyond belief," pointing to the surrounding room, "but I'm sure glad ta meet ya."

"Likewise." James smiled.

"James, this is my brother Weld, from America."

"Oh! Oh yes. Of course! I'm sorry. I did not recognize your name. When did you dock?"

"I got in today. I didn't have your home address so I hired a rig and had them take me to Arlton's. Happily Jenny was there in a meeting," Weld explained.

As always Weld was gregarious, friendly and happy to be alive. James felt they were going to be great friends.

Weld entertained them with stories of his travels and the Bar-X-Z ranch, where he had spent the last year plus. He laughed at himself learning and then teaching Gilly to drive.

"What part of town would a cowpoke like me find fiddle music and country folk?" Weld inquired.

"Well I do not believe you will find many places that are like American entertainment places" Jenny offered.

"Oh I don't know. I think I may know what you are looking for and where to find it," James stated. "Tomorrow I'll drive you around and point out areas you may enjoy visiting."

Jenny raised her eyebrows looking from one to the other. James laughed saying, "I've never been inside any of the establishments but

I know a few people from America, and I've been told they play American country and have American dances."

Weld said, "That is just what I need people who know where I can seek a job and horses to ride and where I might meet a pretty lady interested only in friendship. I'm not in the market for any kind of close relationships. I won't be around here long. I've got a lot of travelin' left to do."

Jenny was up and gone before James called for Weld to start their tour of London. "Good morning!" Weld said. "What's for breakfast?"

"We will stop by the dining room and choose what we like," James offered.

"Ya mean we just say what we want and someone brings it ta ya?"

"Something like that," James said.

There was a hasher of bacon, eggs, English biscuits, rice, milk, tea, jams, jellies and fruit. "If you would care for something more just tell Ben, our server and they will bring it right out."

"Nope, I believe this will do just fine," Weld laughed. He took six eggs, six strips of bacon, a bowl of rice with cream, sugar and sliced peaches and a tall glass of milk which was refilled at least once. "Do we have regular bread?" he inquired.

"Yes, of course." James motioned to Ben to bring Weld some bread. James was amazed at the amount of food Weld put away. He could only hold tea and biscuits.

Weld had so much energy he was raring to go. He whistled and sang as he waited for the man to bring the motor carriage. He walked back and forth looking at the well cropped grounds. Every place was spic and span but it looked cold, impersonal and stiff. "I hope Jenny likes it here. I'd hate to be stuck here for long," he thought.

Weld missed Spike and he worried over Harve, he missed the cowhands too.

He hoped this trip would prove exciting. After completing his visit here he intended to go to Paris if he could find a job and make some money. Here at least he could understand about half of what the people were talking about. In Paris he could understand none of the language. But he had to go. If he didn't he would always wonder what Paris was like.

Weld went into a small pub with a drawing of a buffalo and an Indian over the door. He didn't know what to expect but he would soon find out if he wanted to stay or not.

The bartender looked at Weld waiting for him to order. "Give me one of those," he said pointing to a tankard of ale.

A tall thin man in a big hat came up to Weld, "Ya an American?"

"Yes I am." Weld said. I'm from Kansas. Where do you hail from?"

"I came here from Texas three years ago and I've never been able ta make enough money for fare back," the man said.

"Is work that hard to find?" Weld asked.

"Well fer me, it is almost impossible. If I couldn't play a fiddle and catch a dance to play ever once in awhile I'd starve plum ta death."

"What's yer handle?" Weld asked.

"Jest call me Slim. That's what ever'one calls me," Slim offered.

Weld made a few more places and met a young woman called Nell that was from California. After a while Nell asked Weld, "Do you handle a rope?"

"What do ya mean handle a rope?" Weld asked.

"You know, can you rope a stump, dance through a loop, that sorta thing?"

"Yeah, I guess I'm pretty good with a rope, why?" Weld asked.

"We had a small act down at the 'Cactus' and our rope man broke his arm. That leaves us a man short." Nell said. "The pay is good we get meals and a room over the club. Are you interested?" Nell asked.

"Take me to the place so I can look it over and figger out if I can do the job." Weld said.

The Cactus, was a reasonably nice place with an American motif. You could eat real flapjacks, sausage, eggs, bacon and buttermilk biscuits daily. On Wednesdays you could get brown beans and cornbread.

Weld thought, "I may never work here but I'll danged sure eat here as often as I can."

Nell explained the act to Weld. There was nothing too difficult to do. Weld was confident he could handle the job. In the meantime he could look around for a better job.

Weld had a great time doing the show twice a night. It was like a Kansas get together on special days. He visited with the people in the audience. He even sang a few songs for them.

Weld got the group to hire Slim to play so he could make it home. Slim tried to thank Weld but Weld just laughed and said, “Maybe I’ll need a hand someday and have ta call on ya.”

James came to the club to catch the act. He really enjoyed the show and Weld’s part in it. Some of it was over James’ head but made him laugh all the same.

Jenny saw very little of Weld. She worked long hours and was only home nights when Weld worked at that cowboy place. She tried to find time to go to dinner with Weld and James but they just seemed to miss each other everywhere. She missed James and knew that he was finding her absence hard to deal with. She loved James so much she couldn’t lose him. She would die without him.

Peg told her, "Don't let your work take up all your time. You have a husband who loves you but men need to feel they are the most important thing in a woman's life."

Tonight she had made arrangements to take the next two days off work to be with James. Hopefully not even Weld would call on them. She had ordered the help to prepare a supper of James' best liked foods served before the fireplace in their bedroom. No one at all was to enter until and unless they were rang for.

She dressed carefully in a new gown that showed off her tiny waist. It was a soft green with tiny pearl buttons down the back to her waist and green slippers to match. She was pleased at her reflection in the looking glass.

James arrived home at about six p.m. and was told to go directly to his and Jenny's sleeping quarters. "Is Mrs. Arlton ill? Is everything all right?" he asked.

"Oh yes Mi Lord, everything is fine."

Jenny looked like an angel sitting in a chair beside a small table with shining silver and crystal upon it. The flare of the candles were flickering upon her lovely face. "Oh what a wonderful surprise," he exclaimed as he picked her up into his arms nuzzling her neck, planting kisses all over her face. "I've missed you darling," he said. "I thought you had forgotten me."

"Never!" She cried. "I could never forget you. You are on my mind even when I am loaded down with work but from here on I'll have more free time. I've handed much of my duties over to Madge, my second in command. Right now we have tonight and two more days and nights."

"Ummm!" James said. "Let's go to bed."

"We can't just yet. I've ordered our supper. It will be here at any moment," Jenny explained.

"All right but just you wait. I'll make you pay for all this time you've stolen from me." he said laughingly.

"Oh I'll gladly pay. I've been looking forward to my punishment with much impatience!" she laughed.

The food was marvelous and the anticipation was growing. "I've missed you also." Jenny said, "I've caught my self daydreaming about our lovemaking when I was trying to concentrate on some very important detail."

They didn't even call the servants to pick up their dishes they just put them outside the door and adjourned to the bed. She began unbuttoning his coat and shirt then turned her back to James so he could unfasten her many pearl buttons. She was no longer the shy little country girl wanting the lamps turned off or at least dimmed. She wanted to see every beautiful inch of him, his broad shoulders, slim waist and hips and he had great legs. No skinny knobby knees for him he was gorgeous and all hers. Her dress corset and slips were in a heap around her feet and her camisole was gone leaving only her lacy bloomers which James slowly removed.

"How beautiful you are," he said. "Every time I see you, you are more beautiful."

"So are you," Jenny swore.

This night was just like their wedding night. They made love all night only better.

They didn't bother to get up the next morning. They just got out of bed long enough to attend to their toilette, washing up and brushing their teeth and hair. They rang for their breakfast that Jenny had ordered the night before and were served in bed.

Laughing and feeding each other taking time for kisses between mouths full of food, James declared, "This is the best surprise I've ever had."

"Me too!" chimed Jenny.

"Oh but it wasn't a surprise to you. You planned it."

"I received several wonderful surprises all through the night," she stated.

They finally climbed out of bed around six p.m., bathed, got dressed and went to catch Weld's act at the Cactus. The place was packed with a lot of people asking for Weld to sing some back home songs, which he did. Jenny had never known Weld could sing but he had a good voice and a great delivery. He smiled and gestured with his hands and body in time to the music. A tall thin man played twice on his fiddle. The people enjoyed his music, dancing and singing along. Jenny saw Weld uncoiling several ropes carrying on a dialog as he worked telling jokes whistling and singing short verses of several different songs Jenny had heard all her life. Weld twirled his longest rope jumping in and out of the loop then twirled two at the same time. Everyone was having a good time.

When Weld finished his act he headed for the bar for an ale. James walked up to the bar and congratulated Weld on his performance. Weld was surprised to see Jenny there as well. She was excited and told him she had not even known he could carry a tune. "You are wonderful!" she said.

The ladies were ringed around Weld. They were not loud they just wanted him to know how much they had enjoyed his singing and roping.

Weld was totally relaxed thanking everyone and asking them to be sure and come back again. Jenny thought, "My brother is a handsome man." She had never noticed it before but now that she thought about it all her brothers were handsome and her sisters were pretty. Come to think again, mama and daddy were very nice looking people as well. All of them looked healthy and clean cut. Not a one of the family ever tried to bully anyone and never would any of them take an unfair advantage of another person. If they gave their word you could count on them completing whatever they agreed to or not to do.

Daddy and mama would have skinned them alive if one of them ever stepped out of line. Everyone had chores to do and when the boys got to be sixteen they worked full days on the farm. The girls started helping clean house when they were five. They dusted, carried out garbage and fed the chickens. When they were eleven they helped prepare food, did dishes, hung out clothes and helped care for the younger children. The whole family picked fruit and vegetables.

Mama Abby always told her brood that, "Idle hands were the devil's playground."

Weld told James and Jenny he was leaving for Paris in about ten days. From there he would go back via Ireland then to San Francisco and back to the Bar-X-Z ranch to check on Harve. He had really taken a liking to Harve and was worried about him. Weld didn't expect to stay in Paris over a month. He couldn't speak the language and would probably have a hard time finding work.

Jenny wanted to give him money to help on his travels but he refused her offer. "Thanks Sis, but if I can't pay my own way I should just go on home. It isn't anyone else's duty to pay for my dreams."

James and his mother Peg, knew people in Paris and gave him letters of introduction to three different families. They could all speak English and were friendly, helpful friends of theirs.

Everyone who had met Weld hated to see him leave but he had to see over that next hill. He probably would never come back to any of the places he visited but he would always remember everyone and everywhere he had been. He kept a small journal of his travels and the people he met but even without the journal, he would remember all.

****

CHAPTER 12

The trip to Paris was short compared to the voyage from San Francisco and had a whole different atmosphere.

Firstly, most of the people spoke French. Secondly, they were of a different class of people. The ladies were very friendly but the men seemed stand offish to Weld. It seemed all of them drank more than he was used to seeing folks drink.

Weld just sang softly to himself or whistled jaunty tunes. When they docked Weld showed the address of one of the letters to the transportation driver and requested they drive him there. There was a lot of traffic and people tooting their horns at each other. The French had really taken to the motor machines.

When the driver stopped and pointed to the address Weld asked him to wait. This house was a nice place but not at all like where Jenny and James lived.

He knocked and a small white haired man opened the door. “Oui,” he said.

Weld felt foolish because he could not tell the man who he was or what he wanted. "My name is Weld Winter and I have a letter here for Mademoiselle Helene."

"Of course," the man said, "Come right in. Mademoiselle will be with you directly."

A tallish black haired lady entered the foyer where he waited. "My name is Helene. May I help you?"

He handed her the letter and waited for her to speak. "Yes Mr. Winter I think I can help you." She led him into the salon, "One moment please." She left the room and returned with a note and an address for Weld to go to. "This is an inexpensive hotel and a man there will help you find employment."

Weld thanked the woman returned to his waiting taxi and told the driver to take him to the Mon Cherie Hotel. Weld went inside and asked for a room.

"Oui, one American dollar a day for room and for dinner."

Weld paid for a week and asked where he might find the man whose name appeared on the note. The clerk pulled a rope. Weld could hear a bell somewhere in the back of the building. In two or three minutes a fat man about forty years of age came through a door behind the counter. The clerk handed the note to the fat man and pointed to Weld.

"My name is Gustave, how can I help you?" he asked.

Weld told him of his arrival just today and that he would need a work permit for a couple or three weeks. "I'm just traveling to places of interest to me and I need work to live on while I'm here."

"Ummm, Well I don't know. What can you do?"

"I'm a country boy from America. I can farm, take care of horses and I've done a little entertaining in London. I can try anything once. If I find I can't do it, I can always quit or get fired," he smiled.

"How would you feel about posing for a painter, you know as a model? You have the body and the face for it."

"I've never thought of it. What would I have to do?" he asked.

"Come." The fat man said heading for the narrow stairs. At the door on the left he knocked lightly. "It's Gustave." The fat man said.

"Oui, entre vous," a woman called as Gustave entered with Weld.

"You have been looking for a model. Maybe this gentleman will be what you need."

"Do you speak French?" she asked.

"No, not a word," Weld admitted.

"Very well, we shall converse in English. Do you have experience modeling?"

"Nope! Never even seen an artist before."

"Well, first of all I'm a painter but also I sculpt and right now I'm doing a life size sculpture and need a well proportioned model which I can see even in you clothes you are just what I've been looking for."

"Ya mean ya want me ta be naked all over when ya do this thing you're talkin' about?"

"Yes, of course. How else could I work the clay?"

"I don't reckon I could do that maam." Weld said.

"You mean you have never been completely undressed in the presence of a woman before?" she laughed.

"I didn't say that. I just haven't paraded around in my birthday suit before, unless…unless…well you know," he stumbled.

"Let's start with just your chest bare and see how that goes. Take your shirt off and anything else you have above the belt. Come, come, take it off."

Weld felt this trip just might cost more than he was willing or able to pay.

“My name is Lizzet,” she said. “What is yours?”

“Weld,” he said.

“Very well, shall we start Weld? You must sit very still. Do not change your position until I tell you to. Keep the small smile on your face as it is now please,” she ordered.

This, he found was a lot harder than it looked. His muscles grew taut his neck ached and he needed to stretch. “When are ya gonna say I can move? Everything is achin’” he complained.

“In a couple of minutes.” she said. “Move now,” she said. “I have some work I can do while you stretch.”

He walked all around her small apartment looking at paintings and small sculptures that left nothing to the imagination. There were full paintings of both men and women clothed and unclothed or partially clad. He had thought that a sculpture of himself naked would be vulgar but looking at these he could see that they were just beautiful pieces of art.

He did some knee bends and bending from the waist. He was ready to continue.

"Will you finish undressing now Weld?" Lizzet asked.

He undid his buttons took off his shoes and socks returned to the seat she had, had him on before and finished undressing. There he was naked as the day he was born and feeling totally at ease. He whistled through his teeth without changing a muscle.

Lizzet called a halt at sundown. The light was gone for the day.

"Where are you staying?" She asked.

"Across the hall from ya."

"Good!" She exclaimed. "Can you be here early in the morning?"

"Just knock when ya want me. I will have ta find a place ta eat breakfast but that shouldn't take long."

"Oh, don't bother. I have food here and a place to cook. You can share my food today and later go buy the things you need and cook here after today. You know we get the evening meal here at the hotel."

The next morning Lizzet told Weld, "You will be standing from here on. I can't do a standing work with you sitting. Just face the same way you did yesterday and don't forget that little smile."

He felt a little shy at first with an almost frontal stance but he soon forgot about Lizzet and day dreamed about things he wanted to see and do. This modeling thing just might take up too much time. He might have to get a different job.

Lizzet took measurements of his body at about every two inches. She had heavy wire bent into the shape that she had him posing where she had placed clay in flat hunks, then worked and smoothed it to the exact size she had of each muscle that showed clearly defined. She had done a life sized drawing of him with lines drawn across every two inches. His arms and legs had been measured just as precisely. She said the head would come last but it had also been measured in the same way. There was a second drawing of his backside measured as was the front.

"Weld, you may have a couple of days off." Lizzet said. "I have to build up the clay on the frame and it will take time.

Weld took in Paris on foot. He walked until his feet blistered. He was like a wide-eyed kid at Christmas time. Everything from the clothes to the food was different. Speaking of food except for what he bought and cooked at Lizzet's was just not to his liking. Everyone had told him the French had the best food anywhere but as far as he was concerned he could and would do without much of what was served here. He bought fresh fruit and vegetables, steak and cheese and prepared them at Lizzet's. French cows even gave a different taste to milk but he drank gallons of it. Fish was another thing he cooked for himself and Lizzet. He salted and peppered it and rolled it in a mixture of about one third corn meal and two thirds flour then fried it crispy. Lizxet said it was unhealthy to eat so much fried foods but Weld kept cooking and Lizzet kept eating.

Weld found a small club where the audience was invited to go on stage and do whatever they could do to entertain the crowd. Weld supposed the customers were country folk judging by their clothing. They were friendly and laughed a lot not at all stiff and snooty. Some of the folks spoke a little English so Weld ask them to see if the three piece music group could play accompaniment for his songs.

"Oui! Oui! They play American music. You start off they will follow you."

That was all Weld needed to hear. He needed an introduction to the people so he could find friendly ground. He started off whistling the tunes he wanted to sing so the group could get the rhythm down. He then sang folk songs from home. He was well received and Weld had a great time. These people were just like friends at home they just spoke a different language. They had families, laughter and sorrow and had to work hard to make a living.

Lizzet knocked on his door and ask if he could come in and pose for a while. She had to get the slope of his shoulders and the muscles of his legs.

Weld stripped and struck his pose. He remembered to show that little smile as he whistled softly through his teeth. He was thinking of the night before and the young woman he had met. She was striking, almost as tall as himself shiny black hair, dark eyes and skin and a wide smile. She had soft looking lips and a come hither look that caused Weld to throb every time he saw her looking his way. Some of the people he met told him Margot was a good time girl and worth the francs she demanded and was not infected. He had a date with Margot tonight. Thinking of her caused his libido to sit up and take notice. Weld grabbed his shirt and said he had to take a minute off. Lizzet had noticed his plight but had never batted an eyelash. Weld came back resumed his pose and kept his mind on other things.

Margot answered the door in a see-through something or other. He could see her clearly everywhere. She took his hat off then unbuttoned all his buttons running her long slender fingers over his body and through his hair.

Later Margot handed Weld back his money. "I cannot take your money. I thank you for a wonderful, loving evening. This is something that has never happened to me before with a customer."

Weld walked over to her and kissed her on the lips, a no-no. He cuddled her and told her she was a beautiful lady and that he would never forget her. "If I am here long enough I will be back," he told her. "Keep the money."

The sculpture was nearly finished except for the head. Lizzet had used a piece of pipe to build the head around leaving about eight or ten inches of pipe below the neck where the head would be attached to stick down into the clay to hold the head solid.

Her fingers pounded and pinched, smoothed and applied water to the clay as she worked it into an elongated ball. Finally it was taking shape and beginning to look like Weld. He had not expected to be here so long, but soon it would be eight months and would probably take at least another month to finish the sculpture to the point where Lizzet would have no further need of him.

On the last day she came to where he had posed for all these months and ran her hands over his body. "I never mix work with pleasure but now work is finished."

Weld had never once thought of Lizzet as a woman. She was just the artist. She was a beautiful woman. No doubt about that but…well he just didn't feel quite right.

"Come." Lizzet said as she went through the bedroom door. What could he do but follow. Afterwards Lizzet said "Don't go Weld. Stay here with me. We could have glorious times."

"I'm sorry, I must leave. I'm overdue in Ireland by at least three months." Weld smiled as he lay beside her.

"Then at least give me one more time." This time it was Lizzet who was the aggressor. She went after him like a starving bear turned loose in a small pool of fish.

She did everything to him that Margot had done and with such feeling he had the need to hold her and cuddle her and whisper sweet words into her ears. He told her how thankful he was to have met her and how she had afforded him the ways and means to really get to know Paris. He told her how beautiful she was as he made mad passionate love to her.

****

CHAPTER 13

Weld arrived in Ireland exactly one and a half years after he had left the Bar-X-Z ranch. He had learned a lot about people in other lands but mostly he had learned all people are the same underneath. They all had loves, hates, problems, money worries, happiness and unhappiness. He found that if you treat people fair mostly they will be fair with you.

Here in Ireland, he could at least make known what he needed. The language most used was English but with a heavy accent. He soon found there were two Irelands and they didn't much like each other. It seemed to be a religious thing. He was told to stay on the Christian side of town if he were Christian and on the Catholic side if he were Catholic. Weld claimed neither. He felt his beliefs were his own and that no one had a right to tell him how to praise God.

He was stopped several times and asked for his identification and whether he was Catholic or Christian. He would always answer, "I'm American and I have no preferences."

Weld noticed the buildings were not as tall or as rich looking as in London or Paris. So many of the Irish looked tired and gaunt.

The green of Ireland was beautiful and spotted with so many rocks Weld couldn't see how anything could grow. Later he found fertile grounds growing a variety of grains, potatoes and other foodstuffs. Cabbage grew in huge heads.

The pubs were full of sad eyed men complaining of no work and no food for the children they called the 'wee ones'. Weld wondered why the men were crying bad times but spending their meager coins on stout or ale in the pubs.

It was a good thing he had made enough to live on working for Lizzet because evidently there would be no job for him here.

"Where you from cowboy?" A slicked up red-faced man asked.

"America." Weld said. "Around San Francisco, California. I'm just doin' a bit of sight seeing but so far haven't made much headway in finding much to do."

"You say you are from the country. Do you like horses?" The man inquired.

"Sure do." Weld replied. "I miss my hoss Spike. I left him at a friends place. I hope he is happy."

"There is a place a couple of miles south of town that breeds horses. You might ask them if they need help."

Weld hired a rig to take him to the horse-breeding ranch. He told the driver to come back for him in a couple of hours in case he had other things to do. "Nope," said Sam. I'll just wait. I don't have a thing to do."

Weld went into the barn where he saw some men gathered. "Where can I find the ramrod of this place?" he asked.

"The what?" one feller asked.

"The head man, the boss." Weld informed them.

"I guess you be wantin' to see me." A red faced, white haired man offered. What can I do for you?"

Weld walked over to the man and held out his hand and told him, "A feller in town said ya might be needin' help."

"What do you know about horses?"

"Well, I'm a farm boy born and bred. I like animals and they usually like me." Weld informed the man. "I have helped with the breeding of our stock as well as with some of the neighbor's animals. I'm not lookin' for long time work. I'm travlin' seein' the world workin' my way. I'll give ya notice before I quit. I'll never just walk off or not show up. That is if ya hire me," he laughed.

"Come on, I'll show you the barn and the breedin' stalls, where we hold the stallions and where we keep the mares. If you be needin' a place to sleep we have that too along with two meals a day in the kitchen of the big house and my name is Tom. The pay ain't much, but here in Ireland right now, well…it's bone chillin' bad on most folks. The boss here is well off so not to worry," Tom explained.

"The bosse's daughter sometimes comes around the barns. Don't do more than tip your hat to her or the boss will have you flayed for sure," Tom warned.

"One of those huh?" Weld thought to himself. "Well I'm sure not hankering to get mixed up with any filly so I'll just tip my hat and turn my head if she ever comes by."

Handling excitable stallions is no easy job and could be dangerous if you don't know how to handle them when a mare in heat is close by. The stallions could kick the side of a barn out in his frenzy to get to her and injure them selves. That is why they are kept in a stall where they could be snubbed up in the center of an enclosure, not being able to reach any wall.

The long breeding stalls had narrow widths with a gate that lifted out between the mare in the front end and the stallion in the back. When the men got the two at the exact spot they needed them to make contact they lifted the gate out and stood ready to help the stallion aim his organ which they almost always had to do.

Tom watched Weld his first time around and saw that he knew his business. He never checked on Weld again after that.

Weld cleaned stalls fed and watered all the animals and curried and brushed them until they shone. He talked quietly to them rubbed their ears and patted each one as he worked. He sang softly in their ears and fed them from his hands.

Tom said, “You’re right. You do like animals and they do like you.”

“No work for the next three days after feeding and watering time. Weld you take the morning feed and Jay will take the evening feed.

That way you will have most of three days and nights to investigate Dublin."

"Thanks Tom," Weld smiled, "I'm rarin' ta go."

As always Weld looked up the real people to get to know. So many were jobless and there was little food to be had. He was invited to the homes of many of the folks and sat in on their music. It seemed every farmer had a fiddle and a washboard they played on. They used their bare hands or picks that fit over their fingertips on the boards. Weld knew a lot of the songs they played from back home. The Irish Washer Woman, Put Your Little Foot, Danny Boy and many others. He sang with an American accent and they with the Irish brogue. He had wonderful times. He would often take a plump hen and some potatoes to the lady of the house saying he was really hungry for home cooking and ask her to cook it up for supper.

Of course Weld got home cooking at the horse-breeding ranch but he had to have some kind of excuse to get them to accept the food. When suppertime came he ate very little, telling them he never ate much that it didn't take much to keep his body thriving.

Weld learned to jig and to play the washboard. It was great. He visited businesses and churches both Catholic and Christian. He talked to business men who dropped by for a swig after work every one was very worried about the way of things and those who could get the fare left for America or other countries that would accept them.

So many of the men and the young boys who worked in the mines were ill or dying, of Black Lung Disease, or other contributing factors. Wives and mothers gathered together as if to gather strength from each other only no one had an ounce of strength to give.

They butchered a beef at the ranch and only kept the best part of the animal, steaks, roasts and tenderloins. The rest was to be fed to the dogs, cats, hogs and even the chickens.

Weld told Tom, "I know a lot of people that would give almost anything they have for this carcass. Do you suppose I could do extra work for the remainder of the kill?"

"Sure, take it." Tom said. "Here, I'll get the boys to help finish cuttin' it up." They cut off every ounce of meat from the bone. There was seventy five pounds of good meat left from the carcass. Now all

Weld had to figure out was how to get it to the people who needed it. He had nothing to wrap it in or haul it in. Tom came out with white cloth and sacks. Wrap it in this and use the buckboard to deliver it. Each place will probably be able to pack in a share until it's all gone."

"Thanks Tom ya have a good heart," Weld told him.

Weld told his friends the truth of how he came to have the meat. He couldn't see tossing it to the dogs or other animals. He said he couldn't use it cause he had no place to cook and it would spoil long before any one family could use it up. I have about ten families I'd like to share this with. Eyes were shining and excitement shown in their faces. Everyone took about seven pounds and started preparing it at once. The people hugged Weld but said little. However Weld knew what they wanted to say and what they felt.

Weld was getting a little antsy for a woman. All the women he had met in Ireland were good girls and Weld wouldn't even entertain the idea of approaching a good girl and he was picky about good time girls.

Weld mentioned to Tom that he was about ready to slip a loop it had been so long since he had been with a woman.

"Why didn't you tell me before? The boys here know some safe girls. They can give you the details."

"How about ya Tom? Don't ya have a girl ya visit?" Weld kidded.

"Not any more. I'm true blue to my Martha"

"That's great Tom. I like to hear when a man or woman is satisfied at home. Someday I hope to find that special one and settle down on a ranch somewhere." Weld stated.

"I guess I better give ya my notice. I've got a feelin' I'm needed back in San Francisco or maybe even at home in Kansas," Weld stated.

Two of the hands of Tom's took Weld to a quiet small club where the lights were low and music played softly some where in the building.

A pretty motherly looking woman met them smiling. "Hello boys," she said to Joe and Carl. "It's nice to see you again. Who is your friend?" she asked as she turned bright blue eyes in Weld's direction.

Weld stepped forward took her hand kissed it and said. “My name is Weld. The boys were good enough ta bring me here.”

“Come with me Weld so we can find out just what your preferences are.”

She turned to Joe and Carl and said, “Your favorites will be available in a few moments. Have a seat while you wait,” she offered.

“Now Weld, what kind of lady do you prefer, blonde, black or redhead, tall, short or medium.”

“I guess I don’t fancy ordering a lady like I would a meal. I would rather just observe if ya don’t mind.”

“Very well!” Blue eyes said. “When you are ready let me know.”

There were a dozen or so women in various states of dress and some painted so you couldn’t see what they really looked like. He knew he wasn’t interested in any of those nor was he interested in those who talked loudly or attempted to flirt with him. He spied one young fresh faced woman dressed in a pink dressing gown which she kept closed as she read a book of some kind.

Weld went to her and asked, “What are you reading?”

"Oh it's just a book about a sea captain and a gang of cut throats," she smiled.

"Sounds interesting," Weld offered.

"Yes, it helps keep things off my mind," she said.

"Would you be interested in seeing me tonight?" he asked.

She got up and held out her hand leading him up the stairs. She was tiny, probably five feet tall and a hundred pounds. When she dropped her robe her body was perfect and she smelled good too. Deftly she removed his clothing examining him for any physical signs of disease. "Are you free of any illness?" she asked.

"Yes I am as clean and as healthy as a horse," he stated, "How about ya?"

"Everyone working here is free of diseases of any kind," she smiled.

She wasn't the usual kind of woman one would find in a place like this. She didn't hurry. She talked about things in general. She kissed him on the lips. Most girls like her do not. She rubbed his belly and massaged his back. Perfectly relaxed he thought, "She is so sweet and delicate. How did she ever get into this business?"

She seemed to read his mind. "I chose this kind of work because I like it." She informed him. "No one talked me into it and I had a great childhood."

Weld just listened and thought, "She is the most honest woman I have ever met."

****

CHAPTER 14

Weld arrived back at the Bar-X-Z feeling excited and eager to see Spike and he also wanted to see Harve. He just hoped Harve was all right.

Weld had caught the train at the junction and took off walking to the ranch. He saw what looked like Black Beauty coming toward him. He stepped off the road to let them pass. It was Gilly, driving alone. He was surprised to see Gillie alone. Harve had always insisted Weld go with her each time she took Black Beauty.

Gilly stopped the car about ten feet past Weld and jumped out flinging her arms around Weld's shoulders. "Oh Weld, I was just going to the mailbox to see if you had written. Daddy has been expecting you for two months or more."

"Is Harve all right? Is he sick or something?" Weld asked.

"He isn't seriously ill or at least no more so then when you left. However he has something bothering him and seems to think you will have the answer."

She suddenly realized she still had her arms around Weld. She stepped back, flustered and blushing. “Oh I’m sorry. I was just so happy to see you, er, for Harve’s sake,” she stammered.

“I’m happy to see ya as well and how ya have matured over the past two years.”

“I am twenty now. I will be twenty one in four months.” Gilly exclaimed happily. “Then I can go to Paris or London or Vienna to study music. It’s all I ever dream of,” she admitted.

Weld climbed into the passenger side seat as Gilly continued toward the mailbox.

Harve was on the porch when Gilly and Weld returned. “Weld! Weld!” Harve yelled. “Come here son it’s been too long. How have you been? When did you get back?” Harve hurled at Weld.

“Just got back today came straight out here and I’m fine.” Weld assured him. “How are ya? How’s Spike? I’ve sure missed ya both.”

“Spike is fine, but a little wild. No one has tried to ride him. He pretty much goes where he pleases. Come on. We can see if he will come in for feed.”

When they reached the pole fence which held the horses Weld gave a whistle and here came Spike bucking sideways and bowing his neck. He came right up to the fence and grabbed Weld's hat off his head. Weld crawled through the fence and Spike brought his hat to him. Weld was rubbing and whispering in Spike's ears while rubbing down his fore flank. Spike stood very still and raised his ears as high as they would stretch as if he were being let in on some big secret. Weld patted spike on his right knee and Spike knelt on one leg so Weld could get onto his back. He then took off with Weld holding his mane loosely guiding him with his knees. They were both happy and glad to be together again.

"Harve, Gilly tells me ya have some kinda problem ya need help with. Anything I can do?"

"I don't know." Harve said. "It's Gilly. She told me a couple of months ago that after her twenty first birthday she intends to go abroad to study music. I can't stop her. I thought maybe you could."

"Naw, I don't think so. She told me way before I left she hoped to use the money her grandfather left her to travel and study music. I'm afraid it's her life's dream and she will never be happy until she tries it for herself."

"I have a sister in London that I'm sure would welcome someone from America and a ranch girl to boot. I can write Jennie and get an answer back before Gilly's birthday. I also have friends in Paris. Not close friends but good people."

"Do that, will you Weld? I just can't see her just taking off for some other country not even knowing exactly where she is going or how to get around." Harve said.

"How's yer health Harve? I saw ya entering a doctor's office a while before I left."

"Aw, I'm all right. Just get a little cramp in my chest at times but I'd like to be sure Gilly and her mother would be taken care of if something was ever to happen to me. I worry about who would oversee the ranch and not cheat my wife and Gilly."

"Harve, are ya asking me ta stay on at Bar-X-Z and oversee everything should something happen ta ya? Do ya think yer health is seriously dangerous?"

"Yeah Weld, I guess that's what I'm asking. I have no one else ta turn ta and yes the doc says I don't have much more time."

"Oh hell Harve, that just can't be true. I have come ta think of ya as a second father."

"Will you stay?" Harve asked.

"Of course I'll stay and do my very best but this just cannot be."

"Come on into the den Weld." Harve said. "I've already had papers drawn up that give you control over everything and at my death one third of Bar-X-Z will be yours, one third to my wife and one third to Gilly. You will draw a nice salary as well. I trust you completely. I trusted you with my daughter and you proved yourself to be an honorable man. Be especially strong with Gilly. She will have enough money monthly to live well but not to throw away or give away to some greedy man she may meet. The bulk of her money will be under your control just as it is now under mine."

"But Harve, Gilly won't stand fer that. She thinks she will have full control of her money when she turns twenty one."

"Well she will be told differently by my lawyer when we go into San Francisco Monday next. No use me arguing with her. She won't argue with the lawyer when he shows her, her grandfather's will and instructions on how a sizeable allowance was to be given her on the first of each month. I was to be the administrator or to appoint an administrator of my choosing. Now I have chosen you to succeed me. Now take over the ranch and ask me any questions you wish for as long as I am here. The same two who brought you here are still with me. Give them a small raise to keep them with you.

They know more about the ranch and how it functions than I do. They both like you and speak of you often."

"Harve! Harve! I just don't know if I'm up to handling such a large sized holdin's and all that bank work. I just don't know."

"I'm pretty sure I'll be around for a couple of weeks or more. I'll teach you everything you will need to know by then. We will need to go to town to the bank and get your name on the accounts and look through them and take down balances savings and checking. I don't owe a cent to any one. The ranch is free and clear. Me wife has her own personal account where money is added each month on the first from the ranches account. If she ever needs more just transfer it into her account as long as she doesn't remarry. If she remarries just put the regular amount in each month. She is a good woman but a fast talkin' dude could talk her out of her gold tooth."

"Ya better put that part in writin' too. I wouldn't want to try to convince her you had told me that. What if one of us dies? What happens to that share?"

"All taken care of son in the papers, it is to be divided between the remaining partners or partner."

Harve spent every day in the den going over papers with Weld learning how to do the accounting of the books. Weld had been good at arithmetic at school but this was a task understanding the income the gross and the net each month. It then had to be tallied every four months and again at years end.

They had gone into San Francisco to the bank while Gilly was at the lawyers and to the lawyers while Gilly shopped. Weld had met and talked to Mr. Severs at the bank and Mr. Donaldson at the lawyer's office. They both took a liking to Weld and Weld to them.

"Fellers, I'm gonna have ta have a lotta help along the way. I'm at a total loss. This just is not my strong point. Harve has had me locked up with him for almost three weeks now pounding this stuff into my hard head. I have copies of dozens and dozens of papers so I'll have them at my fingertips at anytime. Still I'm as scared as a rabbit bein' chased by a dog." Weld stated.

Harve looked as though he had, had a thousand pounds lifted off his shoulders and Weld looked as if it had landed squarely onto him.

All the hands were told Weld had agreed to take on the running of the ranch. I'd like for all of you to help him as much as you can. He starts immediately."

They all came to where Weld stood and they shook his hand and patted him on the back. "We are with you," they all said.

Weld as ever whistled and sang but the music was a little tense sounding and he had trouble sleeping too. He was remembering Harve had instructed him to move into the big house after he was gone so Weld could protect the women. Women were just not safe living alone. He would also take his meals with the ladies. They had two servants to wait on them and they would do the same for Weld. They had been with Harve for twelve years and were mentioned in his will for a thousand dollars each.

Weld worried that the ladies might not want him living in the house with them. Then what?

It was two and a half months after Weld had returned from Ireland when Harve told Weld to gather his things up and move into the big house. A room had all ready been prepared for him. It was a large airy room with lots of light from the oversized windows. There were light grey drapes that pulled back to let the sun in or closed to keep the sun out. The bed was huge with a headboard halfway to the ceiling. A highboy was there for his clothes with a nightstand beside the bed. There was a glassed in book case with books on anything from having babies to running a ranch. There were books on horses, cattle, gardening, sewing, history, cooking, medicine and so much more. Next to that, stood a double sized chiffonier.

"My! My! What a big room for me and my two changes of clothes," he said to him self and laughingly said the same to Harve the next day.

"We'll have to do something about that." Harve said. We can't have our head- man having no clothes. Tomorrow we will go to town and get everything you may need.

"Harve, I wasn't implying a need for anything, I just thought it funny." Weld said.

"I know you didn't. I've been wondering how to broach the subject to you. Just pick out anything you want or need and charge it to the ranch account."

Weld got half a dozen shirts and trousers to match, seven underwear, a dozen pair of socks and ten neckerchiefs. He got a pair of work boots and a dress pair, along with a dress jacket and a sheepskin lined heavy winter work coat. Every time Weld ordered one of anything, Harve added six more. Harve threw in two belts with silver buckles and three dress bolo ties and seven pair of their best long johns. Harve also bought Spike a silver mounted bridle and a fine new saddle and saddle blanket.

He wanted Weld to have all these things before he died so people wouldn't say he was using money for his own grandiousment. He wanted everything to go smooth for all of them and he knew his time was very short now. The doctor had told him he had maybe a month left. Harve wasn't sad. He had gotten everything and everyone taken care of including Gilly. The lawyer had explained to her, her grandfather's instructions as to what she would receive each month. There was enough to last her till she was a very old lady the way it was invested. "The amount is set. You cannot get more than the funds afforded per month. Make sure you budget yourself accordingly."

Gillie did not discuss what the lawyer had told her. No one asked her but she was unusually quiet these days.

One Thursday morning Harve did not come down for breakfast. When cook went up to see if he wanted breakfast brought to him he was asleep smiling, so she backed out of the room. She would just wait for him to come down. She spoke to Gladys Harve's wife, who went up to check on Harve. She touched his forehead it was cold so were his face and hands. "Oh Blessed Mother." She uttered and had Harold the handy man to go get Weld.

When Weld checked Harve he knew he was gone and Harve looked so happy. Weld felt as though the weight of the world had just landed on his shoulders. He didn't really know how to go about reporting a death. He would ask the cook.

"I think we are supposed to report some place but I don't know where or to whom," she said.

Weld asked the ranch hands and Jake told him he would go into town and report and find out about what all had to be done. Weld told them to take Harve's motor car and to hurry back.

When he reentered the house Gladys was bathing Harve and had clothes laid out to dress him.

He had been dead long enough that rigor mortis was beginning to set in. "He has to be dressed at once," Gladys said, "Or we won't be able to get the clothes on him."

Weld swallowed and asked what he could do. "Put his underclothes and his trousers on him while I try to get his shirt on him."

Weld was amazed at how calm and efficient Gladys was. "She must have had a great deal of experience at this somewhere along the line." Weld thought.

Gilly had not made an appearance. Weld didn't know if she had been told or not. He certainly didn't want to tell her.

People came from miles around. Harve had been a well loved man and greatly respected. He had advised most of the people of his appointment of Weld as his successor along with pertinent information concerning the ranch. He had asked many of the men to help Weld whenever he needed it. "He is young and has a lot to learn but you will never find a more honest man anywhere. I'm entrusting everything I own to him including my wife and daughter.

****

CHAPTER 15

Three weeks after the funeral Gladys told Weld that she and Gilly were going to London for awhile then maybe to Paris or Vienna to seek out music schools for Gilly. With her allowance combined with Gilly's they would do quite nicely.

"Harve explained the financial end to me and I agree one hundred per cent." Gladys said. "I have never spent much of my allowance so I have a good deal of my own money. I trust you just as Harve did. You will take care of everything, I know. I won't worry a moment."

Weld said, "I have a sister and some friends in London. May I give you a letter to my sister along with her address both at her shop and at her home?"

"That would be nice." She said. "We won't know a soul. I expect to be quite lonely."

Weld wrote Jenny about Harve and his own promise to oversee the ranch and look out for Harve's wife and daughter. "I would appreciate it greatly if you would introduce them to some nice people and have them to your house as often as you can."

He then fashioned a letter to Lizzet and a couple of other people in case they did go to Paris. He did not know any one in Vienna so could be of no use there.

"Mrs. Mosny, please drop me a line as often as you can. I'm going to worry over the two of you." Weld confessed.

While he was writing he wrote to his mother and family telling them all about his travels the past two years and how he had ended up in charge of the Bar-X-Z and held one third ownership in the ranch. He told them Mrs. Mosny and Gilly were going to sail for London the coming Tuesday. He felt as though he was being run over by a train.

"I guess I'm glad Mrs. Mosny and Gilly will be gone for awhile. I need time to learn everything needed to be known to run a huge place like this. If I make a mistake, maybe I can fix it before they even find out I made it."

"Tell all the family hello for me and to write. How are all the newly married couples doing? I hope they are all happy and prospering. Are there any babies yet? No I haven't found the right one yet and mama, I will never take advantage of a good girl I promise." Love Weld.

****

CHAPTER 16

It was round up time and everyone had six different things they had to do at the same time. Weld hired on two extra hands for round up that were approved by Slade and Jake. Hundreds of cattle were pushed out of the brush and corralled. Brands were checked and calves were branded. Slade and Jake would drive the cattle to the stockyards in San Francisco where they would be bid upon and purchased by large companies. When sold, the money would be deposited into the bank and Mr. Severs would credit the Bar XZ account. It was so much simpler since the railroad had come in. The cattle were hauled much faster by train then by trying to herd the hundreds of miles, losing a lot of them before they got to where they needed to be.

Weld thought, "Next year, I'm gonna see if we can't make a deal with the buyers ta come ta the junction ta bid on the cattle and have the train load them on right there."

He could have holding pens built right on Bar-X-Z land that was adjacent to the railroad property where the trains always stopped for water.

Weld ordered up a big feed and music for the hands for as soon as Slade and Jake got back. He invited the surrounding ranchers to come and bring their families. A square board floor was built to dance on and to place chairs for the musicians to sit.

Huge buckets of lemonade and milk were available. A whole cow was being cooked on a spit. There were also mashed potatoes, green beans and fresh baked bread along with numerous pies and cakes of every kind.

The boys got in just in time to enjoy everything. Everybody was having a good time and looked happy. Many of the unmarried ladies looked Weld over. Ummm nice to look at and friendly too but not too friendly. Weld tried to dance with every lady there at least once. He showed no preference for any of them. His happy outgoing demeanor just made everyone feel special.

Weld had a great time. He sang a few songs with the boys and danced a jig or two. He was so easy to like everyone hated to go home. He shook hands with so many folks his hand ached but his smile was ever apparent.

"Thanks to ya all fer comin'. Maybe we can do it again soon." he said.

All the hands were happy. They had all had a good time and had all received bonuses for a job well done.

It was about time Weld found himself a lady friend. He liked all the cowhands, but he craved some one to hold and whisper sweet nothings to. He had to be very careful now because some ladies might get the wrong idea and make a fuss. He really didn't like going to good time girls but he could not afford a serious relationship.

Weld bumped into a lovely little lady at the bank and asked Mr. Severs who she was.

"I think she is the widow who came to town a few months ago. She opened up that dress shop next to the general store. She seems like a nice enough woman but I really don't know."

Weld wondered how he might meet her as he headed to the small eating establishment across the street. Just inside the door he saw her again. She was sitting in a chair by a table that faced the window. Weld took the table next to her.

"I think I ran into you at that bank. May I apologize?" Weld flashed his best smile.

"Ummm, I think it was I who ran into you" she offered.

"I'll forgive you, if you will forgive me."

"I think that is a good deal Mister???"

"Weld, my name is Weld. What is yours?"

"Call me Dottie."

"Would it be too forward of me to ask to share your table?" he asked.

"Yes it would be forward but please join me Weld."

"Can you recommend any thing special?"

"Not really. I seldom eat out and then it's mostly tea and toast. The coffee smells good but I've never tried it." Dottie said.

The waiter came to take their order. Weld ordered, "Steak with potatoes and gravy, hot coffee and a tall glass of milk topped off by a big piece of that chocolate cake I see over there. Dottie, may I buy ya dinner?"

She hesitated a moment, then said, “Yes. I’ll have a steak and one egg please.”

“Is that all ya can eat?”

“No, I could eat a bear but I’d gain ten pounds.”

“Women, always worrying about gaining a little weight. I eat like a bear and never gain an ounce.”

She was easy to talk to laughing easily and enjoying her meal. She didn’t pick at her food. She ate quickly. “I must get back to the shop,” she said. “I have two customers coming in at twelve thirty p.m. Thanks so much for the dinner. You must come to my house for dinner soon. Thanks again.”

Weld watched her walk down the street to her shop. She looked great from behind as well as from the front. He hoped and intended to see her again.

Weld was working getting the deal through with the buyers and the railroad so far with little headway. He would keep at it until he found that he absolutely could not sway them or he would convince them and start building the holding pens. He was forced to spend more time in town now in order to see the beef and the railroad people. Twenty miles into town wasn't like it was before the motor vehicle came along but round trip took over four and a half hours, making it more practical to just stay at the hotel and him being able to see Dottie didn't hurt a bit.

He had found out Dottie had been married for five years, unhappily so. Her husband had died of a stroke leaving her with a mountain of debts and no way to pay them. She had sold their home and paid off the debts leaving her without funds and like most all women, knowing nothing about making a living.

A woman named Jane hired her to help in her dress making business. There Dottie learned how to run a business and how to sew quality clothes.

After two years Dottie struck out on her own taking only the amount of orders she knew she could produce on time.

She stocked and sold ready to wear dresses and under garments along with hand made, tailored things.

Tonight Weld was having dinner at six p.m. at Dottie's place in back of the dress shop. He was excited and looking forward to getting better acquainted with Dottie.

When he arrived she met him at the door in a crisp full, skirted dress from right off the rack in her store. It fitted as if it had been made for her.

Weld handed her a nosegay of violets. "To match your eyes," he told her.

"It's been a very long time since I've received flowers. Thank you so much," she said, leaning forward and kissing his cheek lightly.

She had made a roast with baked potatoes, gravy, green beans and carrots. It was delicious as was the cream pie afterwards. Weld ate so much he felt stuffed. It would take some time for the food to settle. He hoped he could re-buckle his belt and maybe get a kiss before he had to leave.

They spent hours talking about both their pasts and discussing ranch life. Weld was surprised at Dottie's knowledge of country living and of running a ranch.

"Oh I grew up on a ranch in Montana," she told him. "It wasn't a large concern like the Bar-X-Z but we raised horses most of them mustangs that ran wild. We kept about a thousand cows and calves plus around a hundred bulls, which we thinned out every three years and brought in new blood. The animals run free range no fences.

Sometimes round up could take weeks to corral the animals for branding and driving to market. Now like here, it's much easier since the railroad came in.'

"When I married my husband Jeff we moved into town where he worked in a general store. I hated the place and I grew to hate Jeff. He nagged and whined until it almost drove me crazy. We didn't know he had a bad heart but it would have made little difference in my feelings toward him. I didn't want him to die but I was glad to be free. The only time he had a kind word to say was in bed. It made me angry and hurt my feelings. I've always been an outgoing person. I love to dance and have friends around and I need a lot of attention. Not just in bed, but also in bed. I miss the marriage bed but I do not believe marriage is for me. I'm too independent. I like my work and being my own boss and not having to explain my every move to anyone."

Weld could see she had, had a tough time emotionally in her marriage. It had soured her on the thought of marriage. That was fine with Weld. He wasn't ready for that himself.

"You look lovely in that dress." Weld offered. Did you make it?"

"No, no, this is a garment by 'Jenny', a supplier out of New York and London," she told him. "I only stock clothes by Jenny. They are pretty, well made and affordable."

Weld was amazed. "Dottie, Jenny Winter is my sister. Her married name is Arlton. She lives in London. I knew she had started an American line but I never expected to know anyone in the clothing business let alone knowing the person selling the clothes."

He reached for her hand in his excitement. She did not withdraw it. Instead she stepped forward putting both her arms around his neck. "Please don't think me loose. I am just so starved for arms to hold me and lips to kiss me. It's been so long." She led him into her bedroom after locking up and placing the closed sign on the shop door.

Weld just held and cuddled her kissing her for a long while telling her how brave she was and how beautiful she was. He had wanted to hold her from the first moment he had bumped into her.

She began unfastening his shirt and loosening his belt. She turned for him to unhook her dress in back and slipped out of it. With Weld's shirt and trousers gone he wore only short underwear. His boots had been the first to go. Dottie stood before him nude, proud and lovely. Weld slipped his underwear off and joined her on the bed. Their bodies were molded to each other. She held his lips with hers. When they could hold back no longer Weld held her so tightly he thought he would hurt her but she clung to him just as tightly not wanting him to withdraw afterward.

Finally the two lay exhausted sated for the time being. She made a fresh pot of coffee and they talked as they drank it. She could not have children but she did not mind. She really did not have that need that most women have for children.

"Weld, I have no other gentlemen friends. Could we see each other once or twice a week?" she asked tentatively.

"You bet we can. I'd love to see you as often as I can but we need to take steps to protect your reputation. Your business would suffer if people were to think we were close," he said.

"Yes you are right. We must be careful, but I hate it. I do not like any kind of subterfuge."

Before he left from the side door they made love again. Weld felt very protective toward her and treated her gently. He whispered sweet words to her telling her how wonderful she was and how beautiful and how he thanked her for choosing him to be her lover.

Weld felt as though he were walking on clouds as if he could almost fly. He was a man that enjoyed every facet of a woman. He enjoyed talking to them and just listening to their voices excited him and filled that special spot inside him. He sang loudly all the way back to the Bar-X-Z.

****

CHAPTER 17

Bob had been the Marshall for four years now. He had, had to bring in all kinds of crooks but had not had to shoot anyone. He had come near to it though when Darcy Hall had tried to shoot him but as Darcy was not the best shot around and had missed Bob by a foot it gave Bob time to wrest the gun from Darcy and hit him over the head with it. He got handcuffs on Darcy before he came to.

Bob had met Minda Lee at the harvest dance and was growing very fond of her. She didn't want him in the law business where he could be killed at any minute but he liked the law and it fulfilled his need to wander somewhat. He always wanted to go just a little bit further to see what was over that next hill.

He wasn't sure just how or what he was going to do. He had been thinking a lot of Sam lately. He wondered what had happened to him and if he was still out in the mountains. "Maybe I will just go investigate," he thought. He liked Sam a lot.

Bob and the rest of the family went to church Sunday morning where he saw Minda. She was being pouty trying to get Bob's promise to quit the Marshall's job. Bob was non-committal. He didn't like anyone trying to force him into or out of anything. He had left home at sixteen because everyone kept telling him he couldn't do this or that because he was too young.

When they all sat down to the evening meal Bob informed everyone he would be gone for quite some time. Maybe he would be gone for six months or maybe even longer. He promised to keep everyone informed of where he was at least once a month.

"Is it Marshall business?" they all wanted to know.

"Not entirely. I just have some left over business ta be taken care of and I've decided now is a good time ta do it."

He packed his bedroll and extra clothes, a small pot to cook in and a small frying pan, a fork and his hunting knife. He took a large canteen full of water, dried beef, some bacon and some hard tack. He didn't forget his soap and towel this time.

Bob intended to take a train when possible when Socks could ride in the rail car. The rest of the time he would ride so he could enjoy the beauty of nature. It felt great to be out in the open with no one to chase down and no worry about being killed or having to kill someone. He had just taken a leave from his work. He could go back if he wanted to. He just might swing west and visit Weld. It had been three years since he had last seen Weld. From his letters though, Weld was doing very well indeed.

As Bob rode along he remembered seeing his friends being hanged and how scared he had been. He remembered his sore blistered feet and the hunger he had suffered. As he passed through Clayton he thought of the poor beaten man, Mr. Moore and of Tom Port who had beaten him. He wondered if Mr. Moore had gotten well and if Mr. Port had kept his word and provided for the little man's family. "I'll just swing down into town and see how things worked out."

Bob went straight to the sheriff's office but it was a new man behind the desk. "What can I do fer ya?" the man asked.

"I was just lookin' fer sheriff Slate. Is he around?"

"Nope! Sheriff was shot in the back 'bout a year past. A tall thin feller and some shrimp of a man did it. We hanged um but it don't bring Slate back."

“Can ya tell me anything about Tom Port a feller around here or a Mr. Moore, a small man who wears glasses?”

“Yeah. Mr. Moore died some time back and Tom moved Moore’s family into his own home and he is caring for the five children. Mrs. Moore died a month before her husband did of a heart attack. There was some talk that Tom Port had promised Mr. Moore that he would always take care of the younguns and that is just what he is doin’.

Bob smiled and bade the sheriff a good day. He whistled and hummed as he rode along remembering surrounding territories from his travels before.

Bob caught a train out of Springfield to the place where he had come out of the forest where Sam had taken him to rest up and let his feet heal. Socks was a bit skittish about getting into the boxcar but when Bob put his neckerchief over Socks’ eyes he allowed Bob to lead him in and to the west end of the boxcar where all animals were snubbed up. They were allowed only enough room for them to reach the hay. Bob had a feedbag full of grain for when they were going through the woods or down the road where nothing grew for a horse to eat. He still had ten or more miles to go to reach the cave. Bob hoped Sam was still there or had at least left a note telling where he had gone.

It was almost dark when Bob reached the cave opening. Not a sound came from the cave and neither his horse nor mule was under the rock ledge. Cautiously Bob entered the mouth of the cave, still no sound.

"It smells stuffy in here. Uncured hides," Bob figured. He lit a match and located a ready laid making for a fire where he lit the dry grass on the bottom of the wood. Fire began to flicker and light up the cave. Sure enough a large pile of stiff hides were piled at the side of the sleeping area. He had evidently robbed some camp because he had a two quart pot for cooking, sitting next to the fire ring. Bob was tired. He tethered Socks to the makeshift manger where hay still lay and placed the water gourd where Socks could drink took out his bedroll and went to sleep. "Maybe Sam will be back by morning," Bob thought.

The sound of birds twittering woke Bob just before daybreak. At first he didn't know where he was then remembering he went out to check on Socks. He was right where Bob had left him. He hadn't eaten the hay and now in the daylight Bob could see why. The hay was old and moldy. He got the feedbag and fed Socks and went back into the cave to see if there was any evidence of where Sam was and how long he might be before coming back.

Now that there was light Bob could see there had been no one here for quite some time. Dust and spider webs pretty well covered everything. There didn't seem to have been a fight or disturbance of any kind. Bob saw Sam's journal laying on the rock they had used for a table. He picked it up when he saw the name Sam knew him by at the top of the page.

It read, "Jim, I know ya wil com back here wun day an I want ya ta reed carful. Ya member I tol ya I no wher a plenny of da stuff in da bag wuz. I gess I'm dyin' an I got no one ta leve any thin' ta, ceptin' ya. Member wher I cud always git tha fish an ya had a hard tim? That's wher tha stuff is. Tak my furs. I showd ya how ta clene and cur dem. I tuk my animals ta da rod an let um go. If'n no body taks em, dey be fine. Dey wuds animals an dey no wat ta eat an wat not ta eat.

Sined Sam

There was lots more in the journal but Bob wasn't interested just now. He wanted to find Sam even if he were dead. He needed a decent burial. Bob kicked at the dried furs and one slid down exposing the skeleton of a huge hand. Bob uncovered the rest of the skeleton. Nothing was left except red hair and bones. He must have been dead for two or three years. He probably died shortly after Bob had left.

Rodents had been after the furs as well. The cured furs hung from leather thongs where animals could not go. There looked to be about fifty hide hung and maybe another fifty uncured hides in the pile. Rats had chewed holes in some of them but that would not hurt them for sale purposes. Bob went about curing the hides making them soft just after he buried Sam. He had not yet gone to the fishing hole to feel under rocks for gold coins. He would leave that for last. Bob worked many days taking care of the hides and reading the first part of Sam's journal.

In part it read. "I bin gon fer six yers. I tink dey don stop lukin' fer me. I no kil man lik dey sey. I try ta hep man. I be gon, no go bak. I tak my muny. Muny be min. I work fer long tim, sav my muny. My granfodder giv much gol coin ta me. I kep. No spend."

There was never a mention of a last name or a place he may have been from but Bob knew without a doubt that Sam was not guilty of murdering anyone and that he came by his money just as he said he did.

All in all Bob was at the cave for five weeks. After he had finished taking care of everything he stayed on to keep Sam's soul company. He owed it to him and he wanted to stay for his own sake.

He knew now for sure that he wasn't ready to marry and that never would he be ready to marry Minda Lee.

He was going to ship the hides back to his folks in Kansas and put the gold into the bank except for about a thousand. There must have been ten thousand in coin in the large leather bag. It wasn't as heavy as one would expect it to be. Those coins weren't very thick.

He had walked his horse loaded down with furs into the railroad station. He crated up his furs, paid the freight and found the bank where he deposited eleven thousand six hundred dollars in gold coin. It was more than what he had thought it would be.

The bank president came out to question Bob and to find out who he was. Bob produced identification and his Marshall's badge. He hadn't quit his job he had just taken leave. He also showed the banker the journal and gave him pertinent information. He had changed the name in the journal from Jim to Bob writing lightly to match the slightly faded words in the journal. The bankers were happy to accept his business and gave Bob a letter of credit good for anywhere in the world.

Seemed like everything was falling into his lap in a grand way. He dashed off a letter to home telling them to expect two crates of furs and some other things. He explained about Sam but said nothing about the gold. Someday he would explain. Not just now however.

Bob turned his thoughts toward California and his brother Weld. He bought a ticket on the train all the way to the railroad junction outside San Francisco where Weld had written was the best way to get to the Bar-X-Z.

Every time the train stopped for water or at a train station Bob got up and jogged up and down the side of the train. When there was time he got a bite to eat and brought back a sack lunch for the road and a feedbag of grain for Socks.

"In one more day," the conductor said, "We will stop in San Francisco change cars and be on our way to the twenty mile junction. There is a big sign that is branded in big letters, Bar-X-Z."

It couldn't be too soon for Bob. He was plenty beat up riding that clickity clack train. It seemed to take forever and the jerk, jerk, jerking all the time was enough to drive a man or horse crazy.

Yep! There was the entrance to the Bar-X-Z, with large branded letters.

Socks had to get his land legs again. He had, had to stand with his legs wide apart in order not to be jerked down. Now he stumbled like a horse on locoweed. Bob let him walk around for a half hour before he even attempted to get on his back. He was all right now though and they headed for the ranch.

Jake saw a rider coming up the drive lane. Something about him looked familiar but he did not think he had ever seen him before.

"Hey Slade! We got company comin.' Do ya know 'im?"

"Nope. Don't think so but he sets his horse and wears his hat like Weld. Do ya suppose he is a relative?"

"Naw. They live way back in Kansas," Slade said.

"Howdy!" Bob said. "I'm Bob Winter. Is Weld around?"

Jake stuck out his hand and said. "Welcome Bob! Any brother of the boss is a friend of ours."

Slade echoed Jake. "Yes, Weld is up at the big house. Just go right on in and surprise him or does he know ya are coming?"

"Nope, I really didn't know myself until a week ago. I just headed to California and here I am."

"Can we take your horse and give him a rub down and a feed?" Jake asked.

"I would surely appreciate it fellers and so would Socks."

Bob undid his bedroll and threw it over his shoulder taking long strides toward the house. He did just as Jake had suggested. He went in and sat down in a huge leather chair put his feet upon the footstool rared back and promptly went to sleep.

Weld went up to bed never seeing Bob asleep in the chair. Around midnight cook knocked softly on Weld's door. "Mr. Weld," she said. “Who is the man asleep in the chair downstairs? Shall I wake him and send him to a guest room?”

“Man? What man? I’m sorry but I don’t follow you. I know of no man sleeping or otherwise.”

“Oh Mr. Weld there is a cowhand asleep in the parlor,” she quavered.

Weld grabbed his dressing robe and hurried down the stairs. “My goodness! It’s my brother Bob. When did he get here?”

“I do not know. I found him asleep in the chair about two hours ago. I thought you had sent for him and had forgotten about him. Then I came back and he is still there sleeping.”

“Just cover him up and let him sleep. He will be rested tomorrow by breakfast. Wake him then please.” Weld said.

Bob was still asleep when the pungent smell of coffee woke him. He didn’t drink coffee but he loved the way it smelled.

He tried to move but he was stiff and sore. Someone had covered him but he still had his boots on and his feet were swollen inside them. He went to the kitchen to find out where to wash up and get his boots off for a while. Also he needed clean socks.

When he reentered the kitchen cook offered him coffee. He told her he would rather have milk. He downed a large glass in one sitting and asked for another.

Cook laughed and said, “I can sure tell you two are related. You not only look and sound alike but you drink milk alike. Weld has a quart with breakfast everyday and two or three glasses at supper.”

“Well, well! Look at what the cats drug in.” Weld said as he hugged Bob so hard Bob grunted. “Where ya been?”

“Everywhere,” Bob answered. “I’ve been back to the Missouri hills and everywhere in between. Say you’re lookin’ good big brother. How’s it going?”

“The best. The very best.” Weld said. “How about your life? How’s Marshalling?” Weld asked.

“I’ve taken a leave of absence. Ya know how it gets. My feet get ta itchin’ and I’ve got ta go.”

“Yes I do know what ya mean. It’s my biggest fault. I get ta wantin’ ta go some place just anyplace I haven’t been. I want ta know other countries other people and how they live and what they dream. So far I’m doin’ all right here because there are so many new things ta learn and ta keep me busy. But someday I know I'll have ta go someplace different but not as long as I'm needed here. I'm trying ta get things arranged so it will not be such a chore every round up. We have good hands here. We pay better than any one else pays their hands. That's so they won't look fer greener pastures and they are worth it. Jake and Slade could run this place by themselves and do a great job of it but I promised Harve and I mean to keep my promise."

Weld had received a note from Harve's wife, Gladys. "Gilly and I have met Jenny and have visited her home. We all went out to dinner a couple of times. Gilly has met a relative of James'. Paul, I think his name is. They have gone off to look for music teachers freeing myself up to sight see alone. Gilly is just not good company to sight see with. She is always in a hurry. She doesn't take time to really enjoy beautiful things. I really like your sister and her husband. They are very nice and so helpful. If Gilly finds what she thinks she wants and gets settled I shall return to the Bar-X-Z."

Best to all, Gladys

Bob and Weld rode the ranch and talked of everything back home. Bob said, "Mama is very lonesome to see ya Weld. She cries sometimes because she feels all her children are moving far, far away. Daddy says, "Mama the birds get feathers and fly away. It's the way of things." Mama gives him a nasty look and goes ta their room where Daddy soon follows," Bob laughed.

Weld told Bob of his travels leaving out nothing. Bob said, "Maybe I better take a vacation and take your address book."

"I'd like ta see the finished sculpture myself." Weld assured him Jenny would be so glad ta see ya but she is always so busy she hardly has a moment for James. But when he thinks he can't stand it just one more second she clears a weekend and shuts out even the servants spending every minute with James so he will last another six weeks. If he wasn't so crazy about her he'd be gone elsewhere."

"They live in a huge castle handed down from high royalty. His father was Lord Arlton, now James and Jenny are Lord and Lady Arlton but never use the title. Peggy, James' mother was a commoner that Lord Arlton had hired to be seamstress of the castle. He fell in love with Peg and almost forced her to marry him. They were very much in love. Peg has never even kept company with another man since her husband died several years ago. They are really fine people. I liked them all and the Paul Gladys speaks of is Peggy's brother. He is a widower with a small son and a very nice feller. He was friends with Jenny long before she met James but only friends," Weld enlightened Bob.

Weld rode with Bob to the junction showing Bob where they were making plans to hold the horses and cattle to be bought and shipped to the meat packers or other ranches.

"This way we won't have to drive them the twenty miles to the stockyards. We have all ready made the deal with the buyers now we have to convince the railroad to load here instead of the existing stockyards."

"You know here in California grass grows in abundance all year round. The animals can graze about all year. We raise two hundred acres of grain and hay every year and I'm thinking about adding another hundred acres for corn ta feed the horses," Weld stated.

Saturday the hands drew their pay and took off for town. Bob went with them. Weld had other fish to fry. He knocked on Dottie's door just after dark. She was dressed in a lilac dress with rows of lace on the bodice. Pretty pearl fastened down the front and she didn't have a corset on. They just didn't feel good so she just didn't wear one. She looked so soft and delicate Weld had to keep his mind off her voluptuous body. As always she had prepared a great meal. This one consisted of pork chops, a mixed salad, sautéed mushrooms, green peas and chocolate cake.

Weld danced with her and talked sweet words to her. He complimented her on her dress and on the food she had cooked for them. He meant every word. He loved telling her how lovely she was. He felt dreamy, as if he were in the middle of a beautiful dream.

Their lovemaking was as always sweet, gentle and loving. There was nothing missing. They had a great liking for each other and respected each other's needs.

Weld always kept her in his arms afterwards telling her how great she made him feel. He was a happy man. He just couldn't help it, he loved women and loved making love to them and making them happy.

Weld had driven Gilly's Black Beauty to town and the boys had taken Harve's two seater so all the boys could get in. Weld always parked a block away and walked into the different places where he had business then he would slip through the side door to Dottie's. If anyone was in view he would wait until they were gone. He surely didn't want people thinking Dottie was a loose woman, she wasn't. She was just lonesome and needed lovin', real lovin', not just a hop and stop.

Weld beat the boys home by three hours. He was fast asleep when Bob came in to chat. "We looked fer ya. Where did ya go?"

"I went several places. I bought ya some new clothes, under and outer, wear. I then picked up Spike's bridle. It had lost one of its silver conchos off the side. I had a drink or two, I ate and I came home. Why?" Weld asked.

"Oh nothin'. The boys say you don't socialize much with them any more. Have ya gone hi-hat or are ya seein' someone special?" Bob asked.

"Every woman I see is special. You know how I always single date. There is too much horse play concerning dating. I just don't think much of kissing and telling. Weld told him.

"Yeah, me too but I'd still like to meet that sculptress that sweet little filly that convinced ya ta pose live like that. I'd like ta meet up with that tall black haired one too," Bob said as he got out of Weld's reach.

"That's different. No one here will ever come into contact with them so no one even knows who they are."

"Oh I don't know. I might just decide to visit Jenny," Bob said. "Ya never can tell."

"They were all lovely ladies. Each was very different from the others. I was lucky ta have met them."

Bob went into San Francisco to the sheriff's office and introduced himself as Marshall Bob Winter from Kansas.

A fat bellied man rose and stuck out his hand. "I'm Deputy Brown," he said. "The sheriff is outta town just now. He'll be back in a day or so."

Bob told Brown that he would appreciate it if he would tell the sheriff that he was staying at the Bar-X-Z with his brother Weld for a time and could be reached there.

Bob familiarized himself with as many places of business as he could. Each time he went into town he looked over more of the city. "This is a large place that's fer sure," Bob thought. The saloons and bawdy houses were the places where the most unruly hung out. Fights broke out and people were shot in these areas. Not much was done about it as far as Bob could find out. Gambling places and nightclubs kept things pretty well under control. They had men mixed with the customers to keep things running smoothly and safely but every once in a while someone accused someone else of cheating and guns blazed. Most were just wounded usually in the hand or arm so they wouldn't be able to manipulate the cards. Ever so often a couple of hotheads would start a fight but it would only last a minute or so until the guards had them by the neck tossing them outside.

Even Bob didn't venture down by the docking and loading area. When the law went there, they had to go in force taking as many men as they could and still leave the rest of the city protected.

Those that worked the docks were a rough bunch of men. They fought with clubs, pipes, meat hooks, baling hooks, fist and feet.

Their motto was, “If you ain’t with us, you’re against us.” There was nothing in between. They had dock bosses that kept them in line to a certain extent. They had become the bosses by whipping every man who stepped up and they had the scars to prove it. There were almost no guns used in the fights on the docks. They just seemed to like the hand to hand battles.

Ships from all over brought in all kinds of riff-raff along with the good people. You just couldn’t tell which was which by looking at them, Bob thought, “There sure are some mean lookin’ fellers comin’ in off those big ol’ ships.” He steered clear of them when possible.

Bob walked nearly everywhere he went. He wanted to imprint the city in his mind. You never could tell when all kinds of hell might break loose and he would need to know where to get to fast. “This sure ain’t like anyplace I’ve ever been,” Bob said to him self.

There were still buildings in ruin from the fire of 1905 and the quake of 1906. There were people digging through the debris. Ragged women and children and dead eyed men were standing in lines for the few jobs to be had. Stray dogs roamed the streets in competition for food scraps. Hollow eyed and crying with empty bellies.

"Damn!" Bob said aloud. "Why do some have so much while others have nothing?"

There were soup kitchens here and there where only a small portion were fed. Hundreds if not thousands of persons tried to find shelter amongst the rubble.

The so-called upper crust took friends slumming so they could gawk at the poor hapless people. They laughed and poked fun at the out stretched hands asking for coins. Always, some dressed up dandy would toss a hand full of coins into the crowd and laugh at them for scampering for a penny. Bob would have loved to have pounded them into the streets but he knew that sort of thing would just add more trouble to those in need. There must be something people could do to help these folks.

When Bob returned to the ranch he told Weld of what he had seen. He talked about the hopelessness of the people their hunger and of those rich hateful excuses for human beings. Some of them must have a heart some compassion or caring for the children suffering, if nothing else.

"Tomorrow I'll go with ya," Weld said. "We can look everything over and talk ta as many City Fathers as possible. Surely a city the size of San Francisco could do more ta help her people."

Weld like Bob, was concerned deeply. They decided that somehow they would find a way to ease a little of the pain of these people.

Bar-X-Z carried a lot of clout even with the City Fathers. Weld made sure they realized he and Bar-X-Z were expecting immediate action and that Bar-X-Z stood ready to contribute, financially and physically to feeding, medicating and housing the homeless.

A very pretty lady drove to the ranch to talk to Weld and Bob concerning the feeding and helping of those in such need.

Bob took a strong liking for Julie. She was bright, caring, out going and laughed a lot. She laughed at the kittens playing with a ball of yarn and the calves kicking sidewise as they ran around the barnyard. Julie thought Spike's grabbing of Weld's hat was great fun.

When they settled down in the den to discuss what might be feasible she was all business and showed great compassion.

It seemed she had been working hard to get the ear of the people in charge with little success until Bar-X-Z got in on the action. Now there was hope of at least feeding many children.

Julie was the daughter of the socialite Frances Smithers, who spent most of her life abroad. She didn't pay much attention to anything or anybody unless they made the social pages of the newspaper. Her father had died six months past leaving Julie a trust fund. It was a monthly income enabling her to volunteer and not have to work with about one hundred dollars over and above her living expenses which she donated to the soup kitchens in the way of food she purchased and delivered every day.

She had learned early on not to give money. Somehow money in and of itself had a corrupting influence on humans.

Weld was glad she had brought out that fact because he had been about to say that he could contribute money from his salary each month. Now however he would make sure that what he could afford would be for the people who needed it and not to those who run or oversee the program.

Bob offered his services to serve or do whatever he could and he gave Weld five hundred dollars out of the nine hundred that he had left of the thousand he had kept from the gold coins he had banked.

"That's a lot of money Bob," Weld said, "Are ya sure ya can afford that much?"

"Yep, it's all right. Staying at the ranch, I don't need much," he laughed.

Julie really liked both brothers. They were good generous men really caring about other people.

"Ya know we just butchered a steer and there is a lot of meat we won't be using ourselves. Could ya use it?" he inquired of Julie.

"You bet we can. Just load up what you want me to take and I'll deliver it on my way home."

"Ya know we also have lots of eggs and some hens that no longer lay," Weld said.

"Load them up," Julie said.

"Err, alive or dead?" Weld said.

"Oh I forgot about that. We usually get them butchered but if you can get them into town we will butcher them."

"Bob, do ya know anything about butcherin' a chicken?" Weld asked.

"No, but cook and her helper do. I'll go talk ta them." He came back smiling. "Yep, she said it will take about an hour."

"My you boys don't let any grass grow under your feet when you get started do you?" Julie beamed.

"I'll get a program laid out with what you intend to donate each week or each month or for whenever you say. That way we will know where the best place or most needy area is and fund that area leaving other parts of town to run different areas. I have six grocery stores that contribute produce each day and bakeries that give breads and many sweets. They aren't exactly fresh but they are nourishing. Milk is delivered each day the farmer has a surplus. Oh I'm just so thrilled. We are going to help so many. Thank you so much!" she said.

Cook entered and said, “They had six hens and five dozen eggs that had set in the cellar for days but are just as fresh as anyone could want.”

“Cook, you are a dear but I’m tired of callin’ ya Cook. Just what is your name anyway and what is the handyman’s name?” Weld asked.

“My name is Valerie, Val for short. My husband’s name is Harold or just Hal.” Valerie said.

“See there! I didn’t even know ya were man and wife. Thanks fer dressin’ the chickens.” Weld said.

“Tomorrow I need ta go ta the city on ranch business, care ta come along?” Weld inquired of Bob. I’d like ya ta sit in on the meetin.’ No tellin’ when I might git laid up and ya would need ta ‘tend ta things.”

“Now don’t tell me yur sick. I know better than that,” Bob stated.

“No, I’m not sick, but did ya ever hear of accidents, broken bones and the like.” Any way, the more ya learn in the world, the fuller your life becomes.”

"Sure, I'll come along if ya want me ta. I guess I could stand some learnin' on different subjects."

Mr. Severs the banker and Mr. Donaldson the lawyer were introduced to Bob. "This is my baby brother Bob. He's a Marshall on leave from his job right now. I'm thinking he may be active around here shortly. He has been exhibiting signs of missing work lately."

The books were in order. Everything tallied right to the penny. The accounts at the bank were all correct and accounted for. Weld told Donaldson about weeding out the hens that no longer lay and the egg surplus being donated to the soup kitchens.

"That's a worthy cause. I'm glad you thought of it."

"Oh it wasn't me who thought of it. It was my brother here."

"Yeah!" Bob said, "But without Weld's permission, I could have accomplished little. Donaldson looked at Severs and winked.

Bob was shown how the tally was done every three months and at the end of each year.

Weld explained that he had made a deal with the beef merchants and the railroad to load the cattle the buyers purchased at the railroads twenty mile junction. "We will have the holding pens ready by fall round up. It will be much simpler than spring round up was. We won't be driving the cattle into the stockyards. I'm building a small 8x8 foot room for someone to stay in while watching the cattle after they are rounded up. It just might be too temptin' havin' them corralled without a guard. Easy pickin's ya know."

Both Mr. Severs and Mr. Donaldson thought his ideas were on the money and told him he was doing a great job.

"I got a letter from Gladys. She hopes she will be coming home next month. She told me Gilly has her hat set for a gentleman named Paul." Mr. Donaldson said. "Gilly has almost given up on the music thing. It was just a foolish whim anyway. She has no voice of any stature and she doesn't play any kind of an instrument. It was just that according to her music played at get togethers at the ranch or dances elsewhere were so boring and she hates folk music." Weld and Bob looked at each other and raised their eyebrows smiling.

As they headed back to Harve's motor carriage Bob said that he wanted to stop in at the Palace Saloon for a couple of hours if Weld had other business to attend to.

"As a matter of fact, I do have a couple of things ta take care of. How about if I meet ya in front of the Palace in exactly two hours?" Weld offered.

Weld hurried back up the street passing Dottie's dress shop never looking toward the building. He went to the end of the street turned left back to the shop. He knocked on the side door waiting for Dottie to let him in.

"Surprise!" he said, picking her up and swinging her around.

"Shh! Shh!" she said. "I have a customer to fit for a gown. I didn't expect you."

"That's all right, I just had a free moment." He crushed her to him kissed her thoroughly and slipped back out of the door. "Ummm! Close call my boy! Close call!" he said to himself.

Weld picked up the supplies he needed and stopped at a shoeshine stand to have his boots shined up. Standing there he found himself feeling bad. The street children could have had a whole meal for the nickel he paid the boy for a shine. Then again the shine boy needed help too. "Guess I talked my self outta that," he thought.

That Julie girl was a prime filly. No hanky panky there. He thought Bob was interested in her. At least he appeared to be so he would steer clear of any personal relationship on any level.

Weld wanted Bob to learn everything involved with the ranch right down to the keeping of books, the bank accounts, the physical care of the ranch and the hiring and the firing, except for Jake and Slade.

Someday he would want to take a little trip to someplace he had never been and he would need Bob to fill his shoes for three or four months a year. Slade and Jake both liked Bob and would accept him, just as he him self had been accepted by them. Gladys would also be home by then to help Bob or the rest of the cowhands.

Without warning, Gladys returned to the ranch. She just didn't like that foreign food and she had looked the paint off hundreds of great paintings and beautiful buildings, but she just wanted to be amongst friends she had something in common with and she missed the ranch and Valerie as well as Hal. The sun was always shining and everything here smelled so good to her.

It was nice to get to see London but it was nicer being home. Everything was spotless in the house and all was in order everywhere she looked. Weld was doing a good job. She had stopped at the bank and at Donaldson's office to check everything out. She was assured Weld was a capable man and took pride in his work. Donaldson told her of Weld's deal with the railroad and the purchasers. She had seen the pens going up. Everything looked well built to last a long time and the small room for the cowhands to sleep in or to just get in out of the weather was a really good idea.

Weld and Bob had gotten home about an hour after Gladys had gotten to the ranch in her rented automobile. She had enjoyed the ride and the opportunity to view everything.

"Maam!" Weld said. "I am so pleased ta have ya back. Why didn't ya let us know and someone would have picked ya up."

"Oh no need. I just wanted to ride and see everything on the way to the Bar-X-Z. I've missed everything about my home and about America in general. Donaldson was telling me about the soup kitchens in the city. I'm going to offer to serve or cook or whatever I can do starting Monday. Those poor people! I don't know why I have never thought of helping before. I guess we are all too involved in our own lives to think of others. It takes a man like you Weld to see a need and do something about it," she said.

"No maam! It was my brother Bob that brought our attention to the miseries of the homeless folks. I was just as guilty of not noticing as everyone else was. Maam, this is my youngest brother Bob. He is on leave from the Kansas State Marshall's office. Bob this is Gladys, Harve's wife and the boss over all of us."

"No! Not the boss. That chore was left directly in Weld's hands."

Gladys did not mention Gilly so Weld did not either. If she wanted him to know anything she would tell him.

"How were Jenny and James?" Weld inquired.

"They are both healthy and happy with their lives. They are both wonderful people. Even though Jenny was so busy she took time out along with James to take me everyplace to see things I would never have even found to see. I have a letter to you she asked me to deliver in person. Just a moment, I'll get it." Which she did, Weld slipped it into his shirt pocket for later.

“How is Peg’s brother, Paul? I spent a lot of time with him. He is a nice feller.” Weld said.

“Paul certainly is a wonderful man and his lovely son Peter is so smart and polite. We had great chats. He has a playmate now. He said it is because he had been so lonely. His father allows the cooks son to live in with Peter now and he takes the same classes as Peter and is learning music and dance along with Peter. They are both lovely boys.” There was still no mention of Gilly.

Bob told Weld and Gladys he was going to retire. He had, had a very long day and was emotionally as well as physically zapped.

“Maam, is there anything ya wish ta know about or anything I can do fer ya?” Weld asked.

‘No, I think I’m going to bed as well. I’m very tired.”

“Again, welcome home, we need ya around here.”

“You are a very nice young man. Thank you for doing such a good job. Good night.”

Weld continued to include Bob in daily routines of the ranch. Riding every foot of the ranch, showing Bob the many gullies where many of the cattle gather so that in round up time they had to be jousted out. They visited the line shacks and the watering holes. In the barn he showed Bob the veterinary room where every farm animal medical aide lined the shelves. They visited the cellar, well house, smoke houses and the canned food dark house. Weld inspected the door hinges the horse stalls, roofs, feeds and implements.

"We do this every month to make sure that everything stays in top condition and repair or replace when needed." Weld said.

The tack room was neat and held all sorts of halters, saddles, blankets, lanterns, horseshoes etc.

The granaries were full of corn and oats. Hay was stacked and stored in the barn loft. Stalls are cleaned every day or more often when needed. Weld explained.

Gladys was humming and puttering around the house finding nothing that needed to be taken care of. Weld had organized the house just as he had the rest of the ranch. Chores were put on schedule and the schedule was followed precisely. "It is much more efficient and less energy draining," Valerie explained to Gladys.

Gladys had learned to drive but didn't really like it. However she decided she would drive Black Beauty. She didn't care a whit whether Gilly would object or not.

Driving in San Francisco was a bit harrowing but she kept her wits about her and met Julie Smithers to discuss what she could do to keep busy as well as be of help to needy folk.

Julie said, "We can always use extra hands. What would you like to do?"

"Well, I'm a fair cook. I sew very well. I make beautiful quilts. I get along with both women and men and I have some nursing abilities from before I was married. I can teach children, reading, writing and arithmetic."

"Oh you are a gold mine. We have a great need for teachers. Someone who isn't tied down with children at home is a God send." Julie exclaimed.

"Then a teacher I shall become! However, I have no idea how or where to go about getting started."

"I'll take care of that part. I know just about where everything is located and places we can use to bring the children to." Julie assured Gladys.

"Today, if it's all right with you I'll take you around and introduce you to the people. Sometimes some folks are angry or combative. Try to overlook it as much as is possible. They are all so unhappy and at wits end," Julie told Gladys. Always try to observe the food contributions. Sometimes it gets carried out the back door to friends or relatives of the overseers in the kitchen. It is the same for clothing and bedding. I hate to have to watch people but experience has taught me I must."

Gladys was overwhelmed at the poverty the squalor the empty eyes and hopelessness. There were women just sitting staring blankly into nothingness. The children ragged and dirty were fighting over crumbs of food. The blackened buildings or parts of buildings made danger for anyone near them. Some buildings had been cleared off and hauled off. Leaving empty spaces where children met to play. New buildings in the better areas of the city were being rebuilt and new businesses were being started. The streets were full of all kinds of carriages but the motor vehicle was overtaking much of the conveyance business causing horses to panic and people to skedaddle to get out of the way. Most of the country folk clung to their horses and buggies, buckboards or wagons, refusing to believe the motor vehicles were here to stay. “It is just a passing fancy,” they said.

Bob went around trying to get jobs for men with children to feed and care for convincing employers to hire these men. “It will cost ya less and they will do a good job fer ya,” he would plead. He went to food processors, grocers and restaurants asking them to save their left over or unsaleable foods for the food kitchens. He was encouraging a lot of people to join in the programs to feed people.

Many people were glad to help but hadn’t known how to go about it. Bob explained to them they must take a hands on position, whenever possible. Donate whatever you have. We need money, clothing, bedding, food and medical supplies. They can use everything and go to Miss Julie Smithers’ office where everything is planned and distributed from.

He wanted to do more. It made him feel hamstrung when he couldn’t accomplish as much as he thought he should.

Weld couldn't spend time on site at the program but the ranch was sending ten dozen eggs and half a dozen hens a week to Julie's personal area. He knew it was going where it should go and being used for the folks who needed it most plus money monthly from his own pocket.

Jenny had written in the letter that Gladys had hand delivered that she and James were expecting a baby in about six months from when she wrote the letter which made it now about three months before due date. She had also mentioned Gilly and Paul. Gladys and Gilly had, had a fight before Gladys had left. It was something about Gilly setting her cap for Paul and Gladys thinking Gilly was not really in love with Paul but was more interested in 'Who' he was. After that Gladys caught the first ship home.

"I don't know the details of the problem but I believe Gladys is probably right about Gilly's feelings for Paul. I just hope Paul doesn't get hurt again. James has tried to warn Paul in a diplomatic way but I don't know if it's going to do any good."

"Peggy sends her love. She really is fond of you and has great respect for you. I sent a letter to mama and daddy telling them of our happy event to be. I really wish I could have mama near when the baby comes but I'm sure she would never leave America, even for a couple or three months.

I love you and miss you. Your Sis, Jenny and James."

****

CHAPTER 18

Jeremy Winter, the eldest of the family was the caretaker to the rest of the brood. He had always had extra duties and was responsible for how the other children completed their chores. Now that he was married to Carly she was added to the group. Sometimes Carly resented him critiquing her work or plans.

"After all, I'm a grown woman with a brain in my head. I can make my own decisions as to how or when to do the laundry, cook or clean and I can decide when I want to visit my mother or anyone else as well," she would cry to Jerry.

He just didn't understand why Carly should get so upset. After all he was only trying to help her. He still told his brothers what had to be done on the farm and when. They did as they had always done, laughingly saying, "Yes Masta! We hear and obey" Jerry didn't get insulted it was normal. "Women!"

Now mama and daddy were going to leave for four months to be with Jenny when her baby arrived. They were taking the train to the coast to take a ship out to London. They intended to sight see every nook and cranny of London and maybe go to Paris. Weld had told them it wasn't far from London to Paris. Abby wanted to see the sculpture of Weld if possible. She just could not visualize Weld stripping in front of a woman. What in the dickens was the world coming to. They were leaving from the Atlantic coast and coming back by the Pacific coast so they could visit with Weld. Abby thought it might take as much as six months before they got back home. She wasn't bothered by that fact. They had never had a vacation or a honeymoon. Once she had decided to go, she was in a hurry to get started.

Abby and Jacob had left their home and traveled by train to the coast of the Atlantic where the boarded a very large ship. Both of them were awe struck. They had never been out of Kansas in their entire lives. There were so many people. There was so much noise from motor vehicles, factories, carriages, ships fog horns and horses, Jacob wondered how anyone ever got a durned thing accomplished. The ship wasn't loud but the throb of the engine bothered them both. Neither of them grew ill as many of the passengers did. They liked the sea air but didn't mix much with the other people on board.

The food to say the least was different. It was beautiful to look at. Except for fried fish, steak, chicken and mashed potatoes, they left the rest of it on their plates. They drank a lot of coffee and milk when they could get it. They lay in the sunshine and they just relaxed. They hardly even thought of the farm they knew Jerry would take care of everything.

Rough weather caused Abby some anxious moments but Jacob seemed to enjoy the huge waves that caused the ship to rock. Everyone was requested to go to their cabins in case it got worse. They didn't want anyone to be swept overboard.

Both Jacob and Abby slept great the whole trip. They loved everything, including each other. This was the honeymoon Abby had always dreamed of. "Jacob is like a young frisky, newly married man. Too bad we can't take these trips more often."

The Captain informed everyone, "We will be docking in London tomorrow morning. You can pack up right before breakfast and be ready to go ashore right after breakfast."

He then gave a speech thanking everyone for choosing his ship to travel on and ask the passengers to choose them for their next cruise.

Abby began looking for Jenny as soon as the ship docked but could not locate her amongst the crowd of well wishers.

Jacob told her not to worry. They had written Jenny of their time of arrival. "If we beat the letter we have their address. We will just hire a conveyance and go to her home." They waited for almost an hour and decided to get a rig of some sort to take them and their luggage to Jenny's house. Jacob handed the driver a piece of paper with the address on it. The driver raised his brows and whistled softly through his teeth. He loaded their bags and got on the road.

"Look Jack at all those huge castles. It must be quite a distance more to get to Jenny's. These grounds look like they go on forever." The driver turned into a gated drive where beautiful grounds were magnificently laid out in wonderful designs formed by privet hedges and flowing gardens of flowers and trees.

"I say driver! Are you sure you are on the right road. This looks like private property of some royal people," worried Jacob.

"This is Lord Arlton's estates. Is that who you wish to see?"

"Yes, Jenny and James Arlton. Our daughter and son in law," Abby said.

They had reached the castle by a huge front door where a uniformed man stood.

"May I be of service to you sir?" he asked Jacob.

"Well I'm not sure. We are Jenny Arlton's parents and expected someone to meet us, but no one did. I gave this driver the address Jenny sent us and he brought us here."

"One moment sir, I will be right back," he said and he disappeared into the door.

A tallish lady of maybe fifty five to sixty came forward holding out her hands to Abby. "My dears!" she cried. "I am so sorry no one met you. We haven't received any word from you. I am Peggy Arlton, James' mother. Please! Please! Come in."

"They will bring your bags to James and Jenny's quarters. This way please. How was your crossing? Sometimes it gets a little scary for me."

Abby explained that the whole trip was wonderful. Neither of us was ill. We loved the sea breezes."

"Where is Jenny? Is she well? How is she handling her condition?"

"Oh she's doing really great. No more morning sickness. She has some swelling in her ankles if she is on her feet too long. James is the one that is as nervous as a cat. He worries over Jenny working too much or stressing her back, etc. It gives my heart pleasure to see how much in love those two are," Peg related.

"What time does Jenny get home?" Abby asked.

"Oh about six thirty p.m. usually but often she has meeting that can last quite late. However I do not believe James will let her stay too late. He takes her to work and picks her up now. He doesn't like for her to drive or to be on the road alone. It is getting near her time and she is getting a bit clumsy trying to get in or out of her motor carriage," Peggy explained.

Abby was overwhelmed by the size and the opulence of the castle. "I could never in a million years have believed that any of the Winter clan would even see a place like this. Now my daughter lives here and Jacob and I are standing in this room that is almost as large as our entire house at the farm," Abby stated.

Jacob was wondering around looking everything over. Why anyone would choose to leave in a cold dark place like this he could not fathom. If you raised your voice it would echo through the halls he bet. Everything was very grand and beautiful in its own way but he'd rather have Abby's yellow curtains and table cloth and the flowered covers for the chairs. Who on earth would enjoy sitting at a table at least fifty foot long or even across the table at one end. Where did they get wood to use in three fireplaces in half dozen rooms? If he took a wrong turn he could be lost for a week.

Abby and Jacob were looking forward to meeting James. They had received only good reports of James. Jenny's letters always seemed to be happy when she wrote of her wonderful husband and how lucky she was to have found him.

They heard someone coming through the hall, talking and laughing. Abby and Jacob sat quietly with their backs to the door wanting to surprise Jenny and James. Now there was no sound. They had stopped speaking.

"Hello! May we help you?" James inquired.

Both Abby and Jacob turned to face Jenny and James saying, "Yes. Can you direct us to our daughter's quarters?" they asked.

"Oh Mama! Daddy! When did you get here? How? Why didn't you tell us you were coming?" Jenny demanded.

"James this is my mother Abby and my father Jacob. This is James, my dear husband."

"When did you decide to come over? How long can you stay?" she asked.

"We intend to visit you and James until after the baby comes which it looks like may happen at any moment," Jacob informed them.

"We want to see everything there is to see in London. We may go to Paris while we are here to see that sculpture of Weld and we would like to visit where Weld did the rope tricks and sang," Abby added.

"We want to see all the great Cathedrals and the museums and every point of interest. Can we get a map of the city that has everything listed?" Abby queried.

James offered, "I can point out most of the things visitors to London seek out and yes they do have City maps but I'll have to personally show you where Weld entertained. It's not on any map."

"Mama, come with me please. We will decide what we want for supper and inform cook," Jenny urged.

The cook looked at the women and offered. "You must be Lady Jenny's sister. You look just alike."

Abby and Jenny smiled at each other. "Yes indeed, we are related. This is my beautiful wonderful mother from America. What do we have to offer them in the way of American cuisine?" Jenny asked hopefully.

"Oh I think we could have steak any kind of potatoes a mixed salad, garden peas and dessert," Cook replied.

"Fine, only make double portions for my father. He has a healthy appetite just like Weld. For breakfast make flapjacks just like Weld taught you and bacon, eggs and American biscuits with gravy. Mama and the rest of us will have juice, porridge, maybe a biscuit and plenty of coffee. Of course James will have his usual tea," Jenny requested of cook. "Oh yes! Always have plenty of milk on hand," Jenny laughed.

"Now I must bathe and get out of these clothes. I'm sweaty, err, don't repeat sweaty. We only perspire here in England," Jenny laughed.

"I miss the easy lifestyle. I miss my family. I miss the food, the weather and the barn dances. I never seem to have a free moment but I truly love my work and I'm crazy about James."

"How do you feel about this, this apartment or the whole thing?" Abby asked.

"Frankly it leaves a lot to be desired but it's the duty that comes along with the title, Jenny frowned.

James and Jacob were outside walking the grounds. Jacob felt right at home with James and a lot better outside than he did inside.

"Meaning no disrespect but how can you live in that place?" he said pointing at the castle.

"Oh I guess it's all I've ever known so it seems right to me. However Jenny sometimes complains that she can only see the light of day when she goes to work. Then too often the fog blocks out the sun there as well," James confided.

"Jacob got Abby out of bed the next morning at daybreak. "Come on," he said. "Let's get going."

"Go where?"

"To see the stuff!"

"Jacob Winter! What time is it? It's still dark."

"No it's not dark. It's just this danged castle. You can't see the outside. James has already taken Jenny to her Job. We have all eaten and I'm lonesome," he complained.

"Oh very well. I'll get up but it seems like I just closed my eyes. I'm still sleepy."

Jacob had made arrangements to be taken into London where he was told they could hire a carriage and driver that knew all the interesting points to visit.

James had given Jacob Atlton's card that would get them into anyplace and would pay for anything they cared to purchase.

James was to join them for a mid-day snack and then go with them until time to pick Jenny up after work.

Abby and Jacob spent the entire morning at the art gallery and would need to spend several days there in order to enjoy the great sculptures and paintings.

When they saw nude statues Abby gasped and said to Jacob. “Is that the kind of thing Weld posed for?”

“I expect so.” Jacob said. “But just look how beautiful these are. They don’t look vulgar, do they?”

“No but I just cannot believe a child of mine actually did that!” Abby stated.

James joined them for the afternoon visit to Westminster Abby which took all afternoon. They later picked Jenny up and she informed them she was taking off until after the baby was born. She had turned everything over to her second in command. If any emergencies arose they would go to Peggy, at Arltons.

James was beside himself with happiness. He had kept himself from asking Jenny to quit or take a leave of absence because he knew her strong sense of self and her need to control her own actions on every level but it had been a strain on his self control. Now he could help her and protect her from herself. She just would not let being pregnant change her daily routine.

"My mother had seven boys and five girls. She never altered her life and I shant either."

Of course Abby and Jacob were ecstatic that she would be at home while they were visiting waiting for the baby.

"What are you naming the baby if it's a boy, or if it's a girl?" Jacob wondered aloud.

"We haven't decided on a girl's name yet but if it's a boy, it will be James Jacob Arlton," James declared.

"I'm honored." Jacob said happily.

The maid entered announcing dinner. They had a table for four set by the window for the light. Jacob wanted as much light as possible. His great outdoors look from Kansas was the only thing he was missing a lot outside of his children. Of course he really missed the sun. Even on cold days at home it usually shone.

The cook always served Jacob, potatoes, greens, fried fish or other meat and often real American biscuits and gravy. Abby ate whatever James and Jenny ate. She didn't always enjoy it but felt that the proper thing was to try to learn to like English boiled stew or their way of cooking chicken and dumplings which tasted nothing like real American dumplings or chicken for that matter. She didn't know what they added but she liked her own much better.

Abby did enjoy the seafood though. She had never before tasted any kind of seafood. They were too far from the oceans to receive any fresh seafood of any sort. They had their own ponds and creeks to catch a variety of fish and fresh water clams also their crayfish tasted a lot like shrimp and looked like shrimp. Crawdad tails, that's what the children called them. They would take a three gallon bucket fill it, quickly pull off and skin the tail and de vein it of the long black cord. They then washed them thoroughly salted, peppered, dipped in batter, rolled in flour and fried. "Now that was good eatin'" Jacob swore.

James liked Jacob. He felt as though Jacob had a deep understanding of human nature. He liked Abby also but as of yet had not gotten to know her very well.

Jenny and Abby spent hours together. They were very alike and spent their time crocheting tiny things for the baby.

Jenny was so big now she could hardly get up from a seated position and forget it, trying to get out of bed without help. She laughed at herself for being so clumsy, keeping a happy demeanor about herself at all times.

Three weeks after Jacob and Abby arrived in London the maid came to Abby saying, "Miss Jenny would like for you to come to her room quickly."

"Is it the baby? What time is it?" Abby asked.

"Yes, I think it is the baby and it is about midnight," the maid answered. "Wouldn't you just know it? Babies always seem to want to be born late at night."

"I'll be right there." Abby said. She let Jacob sleep. Men were of little help at these times.

Jenny was doubled up in that huge bed. A second smaller bed was being prepared in the birthing room of the palace. The doctor and nurses were already there making sure everything was in readiness.

Jenny let out a loud moan and James almost collapsed. "Can't you do something? She is in pain. Help her!" he demanded.

Abby took James by the elbow and showed him out the door. “She will be fine James. Wait downstairs please.”

James was reluctant to leave but he did. “What if she needs me? She may call for me. What if I don’t hear her?” The butler assured James he would inform him if any word was heard.

It was almost daylight when Jenny delivered a seven and a quarter pound baby boy. James heard the baby cry and took the stairs at a run. He went directly to Jenny where she lay back in their huge bed. She was smiling but looked very tired as James held her close and whispered love words in her ears.

“I was so worried my darling. I kept asking about you but all they would tell me is everything is going well, Jenny and the baby are fine,” James complained.

Jenny smiled wanly telling James she loved him and said she wanted to see the baby.

“Yes! Where is the baby? Where is my son?” James asked.

He had forgotten all about the baby. His concern had been for Jenny. Now that he knew she was doing well he was eager to see his son.

Little James Jacob was yelling at the top of his lungs and kicking his tiny feet while trying to get his fist into his mouth.

James had such a surge of love and protectiveness he nearly cried. He held his son gingerly in his arms looking into his face.

"He is so beautiful. Look at him! He is wonderful! He is my son!" James informed everyone.

"Our son, dear! Our son!" Jenny smiled.

"Of course, he is our son, yours and mine. He is perfect, absolutely perfect."

Jenny could not stay awake another moment. Everyone except the nurse quietly left. James still held his son.

"Sir, we must feed the baby" the Nanny said to James.

Haltingly James released little James Jacob to the Nanny. He watched sadly as they disappeared into the nursery.

Abby didn't want to leave Jenny and the baby for all of the first week so Jacob and James spent time riding horses and Jacob learned to drive. He practiced driving on the right side of the pathway instead of the left because back in America they drive on the right side. He didn't want to learn wrong for the streets at home. He thought he would invest in a horseless carriage when he returned home. He could save hours each trip into town or visiting his children in their homes and not worry about the animals needing fed or watered while he visited. He wanted Abby to learn to drive as well. It wasn't crowded at home on the country roads and it was just like guiding a horse. If you pull right a little it went right, pull left and you went left. The hard thing was to not getting excited and yanking it too far either way and stopping it could take some getting used to as well.

The baby was ten days old when Abby and Jacob decided to go to Paris. They packed one garment trunk that would hold two changes of clothes each and took the addresses Jenny had given them to Lizzet's shop.

They figured the fat man Weld had told them about at the hotel could tell them how to get about and see Paris. They were only to stay one week until the next ship left back for London.

Jacob held up his hand to a conveyance driver who stopped for them. Pointing to the address on the paper he handed the driver he said, "I speak no French."

"I speak a little English," the driver informed them.

"Good!" Jacob said. "We are from America. My son Weld was here a year or so ago and posed for Miss Lizzet. That is where we want to go first."

The driver pulled up in front of the hotel picked up their bag and headed for the door.

"We may not be able to get a room here so don't leave too soon." Jacob told the driver.

"Oh you can get a room. It is the off season for tourists. There are many empty rooms now," assured the driver.

When they reached the desk they were met by a small be-speckled man. "Oui!" he said.

The driver told him, "These are Americans from Kansas. Their son stayed here some time ago. He posed for Mademoiselle Lizzet. His name was Weld Winter."

"Oui, oui! I remember Monsignor Weld. He was a very fine gentleman."

The driver informed Abby and Jacob, "This man knew Weld an held him in high esteem."

‘Is Miss Lizzet still here?” Jacob inquired.

‘Oh oui! Mademoiselle is in now. It’s the door at the top of the stairs on the left. Would you like the same room Weld had just across the hall from Mademoiselle Lizzet?”

“Yes. That would be fine,” Abby said.

Jacob made arrangements with the driver to pick them up around ten a.m. for a sightseeing tour.

The driver handed the trunk off to the counter man saying, “Please introduce them to Lizzet.” To which the man nodded yes.

He motioned to Abby and Jacob to follow him up the stairs where he opened the door to their room and gave them the key, leaving their trunk.

Again he had them follow him, this time to Lizzet’s door He knocked, “Oui! Entre.” Opening the door he drew them into Lizzet’s studio.

He spoke in French to Lizzet for a moment until she said, “But of course you are Weld’s parents. He looks like you Mr. Winter. Weld is a fine person.”

Abby spoke up. “We came to see the sculpture Weld posed for. May we see it?”

“Oh oui! But you will have to visit the Grande Hotel that commissioned the work. It is very beautiful and I am told it draws quite a crowd. There are many life-sized sculptures there but he is the favorite. I think I was able to catch the very soul of Weld. He is such a sweet wholesome man everyone who got to know him loves him. We all miss him greatly.” Lizzet informed them.

“Where is this hotel located?” Abby wanted to know.

“Just ask any driver or guide. They will know.” Lizzet said. “Madam, would you pose for me for a portrait?”

“With my clothes off? I should say not!”

“No, no, fully clothed. You have that same look about you that Weld has. I would paint you in peasant clothes. It will be beautiful,” Lizzet swore.

Jacob stood smiling, waiting for Abby to refuse but she did not refuse. “We have only one week here in Paris. Will that be enough?”

“No, not long enough to finish a portrait. But I can sketch and measure your face and hands along with your head. I can fill in the rest from memory. You have a clear lovely complexion and beautiful eyes. The clothing hides everything else and I can put them together anytime."

"We have come to see the city so I must have at least part of each day to accompany my husband," Abby explained.

"It will be fine. I work very fast on sketches. What takes time is applying the paint and waiting for it to dry before I can put on other colors or shades." Lizzet informed Abby.

Abby was looking over Lizzet's paintings and sculptures. They really were beautiful both the paintings and sculptures. Over in the corner she spied drawings of Weld. You couldn't confuse him with anyone else even in a sketch.

"Why do you keep these?" Abby asked Lizzet.

"Oh I think maybe he will come back someday and I will paint him."

"You can't paint him from memory the way you said you would do me."

"Not and do him justice," she mused. "It's a feeling I must capture as well as the features. He is elusive just like quicksilver. One must move fast to catch his aura.

Jacob had formed a friendship with Jim, the guide. Jim was just a country boy who came to town to make his way only to find there were many for every position so he bought himself a horse and carriage. Now the new fangled motor carriages were about to put him out of business. Now he was all right, but in a couple of years, well, au revoir.

By the fourth day Jacob had about looked over everywhere but he wanted to see the Can-Can danced. It was now or never. He didn't intend to leave America ever again. It had been interesting he had enjoyed seeing how the other half lived but he was now ready for home.

Abby agreed to go to the Follies Bergere, "But if they are too crude, I'm leaving."

It was wonderful, the music the dancing those costumes and the paintings on the walls. The ladies were pretty. A bit raucous but nothing she wouldn't do herself if she could. You don't raise a house full of boys and stay a prude.

Jacob was having the time of his life. "Mama, I'm gonna buy one of those costumes and take it home so you can dance the Can-Can for me," he laughed.

"Bring it on!" she said. "I can outdo any one of the girls." she pointed to the stage laughing.

The fifth day Lizzet dressed Abby in peasant clothes and had her continue the pose she held each day. While Lizzet sketched and measured they spoke of Weld and how at first he said he couldn't disrobe fully until he looked over her other work. Then he had just slipped out of all his clothes as if he had done it all his life.

Today they were going to the hotel to view Weld's statue. Abby just hoped she wouldn't show it if she were flustered. "Jacob, do not leave my side!" she ordered as they drew up in front of the huge lavish building that housed the hotel and Weld's sculpture.

They entered hesitated, looked around and joined a group of people in front of a, Beautiful piece of work by Lizzet.

"She has outdone herself on this one," they were saying.

"He looks as though he could just take off and walk," one man said.

"Yes, look at that secret little grin she has caught."

"How beautiful!" a woman breathed.

Abby and Jacob worked themselves closer to the statue. Tears came into Abby's eyes. "Oh Jacob, look how beautiful our son is."

Someone heard them say 'our son' and gathered around them, "Where is your son? Where are you from? What do you think of the sculpture? Does it really look like him?" Etc. etc.

"We are from America," Jacob offered. "Yes it looks just like my son. We also think it is beautiful."

The crowd followed them outside still asking questions. Jacob told the driver to drive on. Abby sat quietly. Tears glistened in her eyes then rolled down her cheeks.

"I'm so glad we came. I only wish we could take it home with us."

We have only tomorrow left. The next day we board ship back to Jenny's. We must leave for America the next sailing date," Jacob told Abby.

Jacob spent a half hour visiting Lizzet telling her how beautiful the work of Weld was.

Abby posed for Lizzet the rest of the day and the next day. She was sorry she couldn't see the finished work. She was sure Lizzet would do it true to life.

Lizzet and Jim saw them off. They waved until the ship was too far off to see the passengers, faces. "They are like their son, very nice people," Lizzet sighed.

Jenny and James met them and they all went to eat at the new American restaurant. They all had cottage fried potatoes, fried chicken, creamed peas, asparagus and chocolate cake with tall glasses of milk.

The women could not finish theirs but both men ate every crumb then they took a long ride over London.

"How is my grandson?" Abby inquired.

"Yes, how is James Jacob Arlton? Has he grown in the week?" Jacob wanted to know.

"You know, I think he has grown. He looks for Jenny and follows her with his eyes. I think I'm jealous," James said.

"I can hardly keep James away from baby long enough to let him sleep. James is going to have him so spoiled he will be a cry baby."

Their tickets were purchased for America. "Everything is packed and ready to load tomorrow morning," Jacob informed everyone.

They had not informed Weld they were coming so they hired a motor car and driver and told him to take them to the Bar-X-Z ranch. The twenty miles to the railroad junction passed so quickly they hardly had time to see the view. When they turned left into the Bar-X-Z lane they both began to become excited. The grass was green and tall swaying in the breeze. They saw the acres and acres of land with cattle and horses feeding leisurely. The lakes were clear blue and the forested land was beautiful.

They could see the house, barn and half dozen other buildings, all well kept. No refuse dotted any part of the ranch. It made Jacob proud knowing Weld was in charge and was doing his job well.

Someone was pointing toward them. It looked like Bob not Weld, but that couldn't be. Bob had gone to Missouri and then was going back home because he had a job as a Kansas Marshall. It was in fact Bob. Weld was riding fence with some of the boys.

"Papa! Mama! Where did you come from? My goodness I'm glad ta see ya. Why didn't ya let us know? We would have loved ta pick ya up anywhere at all. Come in, come in. I'm just flustered. I can't believe ya are here. Wait until Weld gets back."

"Gladys, where are ya? Could ya come and meet my parents?

No one answered so he went into the kitchen asking Valerie, "Where is Ms. Gladys?"

"She is down at the barn de-nesting some old setting hens. She isn't ready for new hatchlings just yet. She should be back anytime. Why don't you take your parents up to Weld's room so they can change and rest up? Gladys will appoint a room for them and I'll get it ready. I'll bring up some coffee and cream pie for now if that's agreeable." Val offered.

"Yes, of course Val. Come with me Mama and Papa. Gladys will be back soon. In the meantime why not rest. I know how travel is so tiring. When I got here I went to sleep in that big ol' chair before Weld got home and he didn't see me sittin' there. Cook saw me early in the evening not even knowing who I was. When she saw me still sittin' there after midnight, she asked Weld who I was and where ta put me. Weld didn't have a clue who this sleepin' cowhand was so he came downstairs saw it was me, had Val cover me up and went back ta bed."

Bob was talking so much and so fast Abby or Jacob couldn't get in a word edgewise. They followed Bob up the stairs glad to be getting some place to lie down for a few minutes. Both of them were very tired. The time difference was catching up to them.

Jacob and Abby loosened their outer clothing and undid their buttons. Jacob kissed Abby and both lay over on the bed. They promptly fell asleep.

Gladys returned to the house and was told of the arrival of Weld and Bob's parents. Val and Gladys set about opening a guest room on the west side of the house.

Weld had gotten back and looked in on his parents who were napping peacefully. He backed out of the room quietly letting them rest.

Valerie put a plate of sandwiches and a plate of sliced fruit along with milk on a tray. If or when they awoke and were hungry they could eat while everyone else slept. In the morning they could all have breakfast together.

It was three a.m. when Abby awoke. “Jacob! Jacob!” she said as she poked his ribs. Look at what time it is. Everyone must be asleep. They have left food for us. We had better get undressed and get into bed properly.” Which is just what they did after they consumed the food.

At five a.m. Abby heard noises from down stairs. She quickly dressed after using the washbowl of water to freshen up. She left Jacob’s razor out to remind him his whiskers were getting a head start on him.

Gladys saw Abby descending the stairs and went toward Abby smiling, hands extended in welcome. “I am Gladys. I expect you are the Winter boy’s Mother.”

“Yes. I am so sorry to have caused an inconvenience for you last night. We just fell asleep and did not wake until three a.m. I haven’t been asleep since then but my husband is still sleeping.”

“It was no trouble at all.” Gladys assured her.

Weld smelled coffee and made his way to the kitchen where Gladys and Abby were sitting at the kitchen table with steaming cups between them.

Weld rushed to his mother gathering her into his arms. “Mama! Mama! It’s so good ta see ya. I’ve missed ya and Papa so much. Where is Papa?” He inquired.

Abby laughed saying, “Sleeping like a bear in winter. He was really tired.”

“You are lookin’ more beautiful every year.” Weld swore.

“Where is Bob?” Abby inquired.

“Oh he’s probably lining the hands out fer the day’s work. I’ve put him to work.”

“What do ya think about my mother Gladys? My beautiful mother,” Weld asked.

“We are fast becoming friends,” Gladys replied.

Jacob and Bob both entered about the same time.

“Papa!” Weld said. Ya look younger and healthier, just like Mama.” As he grabbed his father’s hand and gave him a big hug.

"Yes we have had a great time especially seeing Lizzet's sculpture of you that stands in that fancy hotel in Paris," Jacob laughed.

Weld blushed. "I'm sorry to have embarrassed you and Mama," he whispered.

"No, no, we were proud and happy. It is a beautiful thing to behold. We visited art galleries in both London and Paris before we went to the hotel. None were as beautiful as yours by Lizzet."

Abby hugged Weld and told him she was proud of him.

"Mama posed for a portrait by Lizzet. She was dressed in peasant clothes. Of course there was not time to finish the painting but Lizzet says she can paint it from memory. She took measurements and sketched Abby for hours. I wish we would be able to see the end result," Jacob said.

"Today Gladys is taking me into San Francisco to the people all of you are involved in caring for. Maybe I can do something to help while we are here," Abby disclosed.

"We are riding today showing Papa the ranch," Weld told his mother. Abby was pleased that Jacob would get to do the things he loved. He had missed the outdoors very much.

The men ate enormous amounts of food as usual, Jacob especially. He was so hungry for good farm fare he ate as if this would be the last chance to eat a meal in his life time. Everybody laughed at him but he didn't care. It was real coffee too and milk that tasted like milk and biscuits made with clabber.

"I'm a happy man," he said, patting his belly.

The men loaded Gladys motor carriage with eggs, chickens, blankets and clothes to be taken to Julie. She would then take them to where they were most needed. The women then climbed into the seat.

Gladys started the machine and drove perfectly down the lane to the road and into town. "My goodness!" Abby observed. "There is as much traffic here as there is in Paris or London."

"Yes, it is getting crowded on the streets now but we are getting used to it," Gladys agreed.

As they went further into the worst part of the city, Abby began to see what Gladys and the boys were talking about. She saw so many tragic eyes peering at them the Hopelessness, the small children with dirty hungry faces. She saw men and women trying to console hungry frightened babies. "We must do something now," Abby said.

Gladys had told Abby about Julie Smithers and that Weld says he thinks Bob is rather smitten with her. “Of course Weld could be wrong about that,” opined Gladys.

“If Weld suspects Bob is attracted to Miss Smithers he probably is,” Abby stated.

“Hello Julie! This is Mrs. Winter, Weld and Bob’s mother. Abby, this is Julie.” Gladys introduced them.

“I am very pleased to meet you,” Julie stated. “Please be seated so we can get the schedule mapped out then maybe we could talk. I would love to know about Bob and Weld of course. How they grew up to be such wonderful men. You just do not find men of their caliber very often. You and your husband must be great role models.

“Thank you Julie. We practiced what we preached but we are so fortunate to have good children to work with. You can do wonders if you have good clay to mold with. If not and with too much sand it will just crumble away.”

Gladys and Abby took the items to Julie’s pet program area and went inside to talk to the overseer of this kitchen. He was so happy to receive the chickens and eggs from the farm because another supplier had failed to show up and they were down to the last few plates of food for the children Gladys was trying to teach. Abby had home schooled her kids through the eighth grade so she was very helpful to Gladys and loved every moment of it.

When they finally started home it was beginning to sprinkle lightly. They would get a little damp but that didn't matter to either Gladys or Abby. They felt good at having done so much for people who have nothing. Their automobile jostled right along amongst all the horse carriages some of the animals shied away from the noisy motor cars but more and more of the horses were becoming used to the horseless carriages as they made way, side by side or nose to tail as the case may be.

Abby had only seen half a dozen or so automobiles before they left home now they were everywhere. London and Paris had about half and half or maybe a little less motor vehicles compared to horse drawn carriages. Only the wealthy could afford those in the downtown areas. Very few were seen on country roads or on farms unless some romantic young man was taking his lady friend for a slow country ride.

The men were all in from the ranch chores. Cook was putting fresh milk in stone crocks and pitchers. She was sending yesterday's surplus to the hogs, chickens, cats and dogs.

Gladys was trying to figure a way to send milk into the soup kitchens. Milk just isn't a food you could keep fresh long enough to deliver it to the city on a daily schedule.

Everyone, talking at once was trying to critique efforts for the day.

Abby was excitedly trying to explain to Jacob the many things she had seen and helped with in the city.

Bob asked if she had met Miss Smithers and if she had liked her?

"Yes! She was the first person I met. She asked about you Bob and Weld as well as an after thought!" Abby bubbled.

Bob pretended to be unaware of his mother's teasing as everyone nudged each other.

"Papa, I heard ya learned ta drive at Jenny's. Are ya gonna buy an automobile when ya get home?" Weld asked.

"Maybe next year or in 1912. I'm waitin' fer that Ford feller ta put up or shut up. He says he will have a machine by then that will go much faster and fer under a thousand dollars," Jacob informed them.

"Ya know I did read about that only last week," Bob said. "Guess I'll wait and see as well."

"Say, tell us about Jenny and yer new grandson. What's his name? Is he healthy?" Bob asked.

"He's a real joy and yes, he seems to be very healthy," Abby volunteered. "He is the apple of his daddy's eye."

Jacob spoke up and informed them, "His name is James Jacob Arlton. Jenny is taking time off work ta get ta know him and him ta know her. James says the baby's eyes follow Jenny around and he says he thinks he may be jealous of James Jacob because Jenny gets more of J.J.'s attention than he does and J.J. gets more of Jenny's time than he does. He had to share Jenny with her work before and he would get discontented when they too often had too little time ta even dine together. Of course he was just pretending about the baby. He's crazy about him and Jenny as well. They have a wonderful life but I'd never be able ta live in that gray dungeon. The grounds are beautiful but the weather is too grey and foggy ta enjoy it."

Every day Abby and Gladys went into the city to teach the children and to take a ten gallon container of fresh milk for the babies.

Abby had wanted so badly to return to her home now she hated to leave. There was so much to do to care for the children and to feed the adults so they would have the strength to look for work to become self sustaining once more.

Jacob however was itching to get started home. He missed his other children and the farm. He was keeping busy on the ranch, "but home is where the heart is," he told the boys.

Bob and Weld hated to see their parents leave. It was so far away. Everyone had their own lives. They were all busy all the time leaving very little time to take off across country to visit anyone.

Letters had been sent telling Jerry when Abby and Jacob would arrive home. They would have to travel by train and then coach then by train again. It was nothing to look forward to. It would be long tiring hours and for such a long time.

The boys held onto their parents not wanting to let them go. They watched until the train was out of sight neither of them having much to say on the ride back to the ranch. Each of them thinking it would be years before they saw their parents again.

Weld took Spike for a long ride over the ranch. He sang and whistled as he rode.

Bob went into town to see if Julie had some place where he could be of help.

****

CHAPTER 19

Jerry met Jacob and Abby and took them to the farm. They talked about a mile a minute all the way home. Jacob wanted detailed information about everything that had happened since they had left about five months before.

Jerry on the other hand wanted to know all about their trip. He wanted to hear all about Jenny and her family and Weld and Bob also.

Abby could not get a word in with the two of them trying to talk over each other's words. Abby clapped her hands as she always did to get their attention. Both stopped speaking and looked at her. "Now! What are you trying to hide Jeremy? Out with it!"

"Ummm, I thought it could wait until we all sat down ta supper."

"What can wait?" Jacob asked.

"Papa, really it's nothing great but I would like ta wait 'til everyone is present. Tonight they are preparing a feast fer ya, fer all of us." Jerry pleaded.

"Very well, we will wait," Abby interposed. "You will wait to hear about the trip until we are all present as well."

They were close enough to home to see the carriages and hear the children playing. Abby was so eager to see everyone she felt like jumping out and running the rest of the way but she contained herself until the carriage stopped. The whole yard and porch were full of people welcoming them home with lots of hugs and kisses. Oh it was wonderful to be home again even though she saw the look that passed between Jerry and the other boys. At least no one was ill or hurt. Everyone was here and appeared to be in good health. Abby sighed to her self she could handle anything else no matter what!

Supper was about twenty minutes from ready to eat, giving Jacob and Abby time to wash up and change clothes. They were sweaty and dusty from days of traveling. A good all over bath was what they really needed but that would have to wait until bedtime.

"First, Jenny, baby and James are wonderful. Weld and Bob are well, happy and loving their lives. Now, let's have the news from here," Abby demanded.

Jerry looked at Carl who looked at Frank and Henry. Jackson didn't look up. "Well?"

"Maybe Carl should start," Jerry offered.

"Well, someone start!" Jacob stressed.

"Uhh, well…I guess we decided Jerry was pushing us too hard. Ya know how he had always been in charge of us boys while we were growing up telling us what we could do and how ta do it. Well, we're grown men now and we know how ta do what is needed ta be done and when ta do it, only Jerry thinks different. We have wives now at least Frank and I do and we need ta spend a little more time at home with them.

Jacob questioned, "Just what exactly did Jerry ask you ta do?"

"Well, it's more like when ta do certain chores. It's like he wants us ta start at seven thirty and stayin' until milkin' and feedin' has been completed and workin' Saturdays, things like that," Carl said.

"When I am here what days and what times do we work?" Jacob asked.

"Uh, about the same I guess, but we didn't have families before." Carl insisted.

"When we hire harvest help what time do we work?"

"Sun up ta sun down I guess," Carl admitted.

"Are the men we hire when we need more help married men for the most part?"

"Yes, I think they are."

"Do ya think ya should work under different rules than the other men?" Jacob queried.

Carl looked at Frank who just shrugged and said nothing.

"Jerry, what do ya have ta add ta this complaint?"

"Nothin'. I just followed yer instructions just as I always have. It just takes so many hours ta complete the chores. I work right along with everyone else, plus I keep the books up and restock whatever is low and I also am married."

"All right, I'll think on this tonight and tomorrow, after that we will see," Jacob promised.

"Everyone gather all around. We will tell ya all about our trip. It was wonderful! We spent days lookin' at the Great Churches and Cathedrals in both London and Paris. Do ya know those Cathedrals were made way back sometime in the twelve hundreds? I just cannot figure out how those building were put up and how they have stayed up. All of them are grey from years of coal smoke. A dirty dingy grey, but they look as though they will still be standing for hundreds of years to come," Jacob expanded.

The very best experience we had, was in Paris where we viewed the beautiful sculpture of 'Weld, by Lizzet'. Mama was at first afraid ta look but after she listened ta so many people saying how beautiful and how lifelike it was she opened her eyes ta look and she cried from the beauty of the piece. She knew our son had been immortalized for all times for many generations ta enjoy."

"I looked over art work in London and Paris and none was so beautiful as my son," Abby proudly stated.

The next day Jacob went around the farm looking to see if everything had been kept up in his absence. He could find nothing left undone.

Jacob and Abby had talked for many hours to to decide the best way to handle the squabble between the boys.

Abby as always understood the differences in the needs of the married boys. After all they had small farms of their own with animals to care for and wives who needed attention.

Jacob argued, "We need the work done right and on time or we will not produce and no one will benefit."

"Maybe we can start paying the boys by the hours they put in instead of a flat weekly or monthly rate?" Abby suggested.

"What about the needed work to keep everything producing?" Jacob asked.

"Hire someone to make up the hours needed," she offered. "How about Jerry? He has the biggest load to carry and the extra farm chores at his home," Abby said.

"Yeah, I guess it's about time each of them had their own home and run it as they see fit. I just don't want any of them digging at one another. We are family and we must always be close and love each other," Jacob said.

Jacob sat down and tried to make a reasonable schedule. It was hard. If he let the married boys off the other two would feel slighted. It had to be the same for all five boys. He called all five of them into the living room an hour before quitting time. He told them how pleased he was over the way they had taken care of the farm while he and Abby had been away.

"I've made some changes for each of ya in the hours ya will be needed ta work also in the days and the pay rate. Your mother and I realize married folks with chores of their own need time ta take care of their homes so if you are agreeable, here is what we suggest. Ya can have every other Saturday and Sunday off. We will start paying ya by the hours ya put in each day. Just let me know the hours we can depend on ya ta be here. I'll hire people to pick up the work ya can't get finished in the hours ya do work. If Jerry still wants the foreman's job he is still the boss. If any of ya can't handle that now is the time ta speak up," Jacob told them.

"Uhh Papa, I believe I'll pass on being foreman. I just don't have time ta continue that. I'd like ta be able ta work my own farm a little more. I'm always all tuckered out and get grumpy at home," Jerry said.

Carl spoke up and said, "It's just the same with me. We want ta get some milk cows and raise some hay ta feed them. I figure the most I can give ya is three days a week."

Frank and Henry agreed with Carl and Jerry. We will give ya plenty of time ta find good help and ya know anytime yer help doesn't show we will be right here."

Jackson said, "I ain't got a wife or a farm but I'd sure appreciate Saturdays off. I kinda like dancing the ladies around, if ya know what I mean." Everyone laughed and gave Jack a little push or punch.

"All right, three days a week it is except fer Jack. He thinks he can handle five days as usual. Boys, each of ya make me a worksheet fer the days and hours ya want ta work so I can figure out how many men I'm gonna need ta hire. Now, is everyone satisfied? Do ya have any more suggestions or complaints?" No one said a thing.

"Abby, I'm tellin' ya, gettin' part time help won't be easy and I suppose I'll have ta be on hand every morning to get everything started. What do ya think about getting' rid of the milk cows, except fer a couple of them and adding beef cattle? That would cut hours off fer the milkin' and feedin' twice a day. Two milk cows will furnish the family with all the milk, cheese and butter we can use," Jacob suggested.

"Of course Jacob, if that's the way you think is best. We don't have all those mouths to feed now. We can do nicely from the milk with just two animals." Abby assured him.

"We can sell a lot more eggs and fryers now as well since we use less than half of what we did. That will offset the money for the milk and cream and without the extra hours we usually pay for milking we should come close to averaging about the same income," Jacob informed Abby.

Jacob put out the word for the hands he would like to hire and the hours he needed them.

By bedtime, most things were in the works. Daughter's in law were happier, the boys were more light hearted and everyone seemed to be more satisfied.

When bedtime came, Jacob pulled Abby toward him saying, "Come here sweet woman. Your husband needs your lovin'. It's been so long, I'm afraid I may have forgotten how," he laughed.

"Oh yes! I can just see you forgetting how to love me."

Jacob undid Abby's long thick hair and watched it tumble over her bare shoulders and down her back. Her skin had never gotten stretch marks as so many mothers did. Her breasts were only slightly less firm than when he had first seen them. She had soft skin all over that glowed in the moonlight coming through the window. He rubbed her shoulders and her belly. She felt that same thrill he had always given her. She waited for what she knew was to come next. Slowly he began to kiss her eyes, her lips and her breast. The passion began to surge through her entire being. She clung to him kissing where she could reach. Pulling him ever closer she cried, "Jacob, Jacob, my sweet husband. I love you! I love you!" as she quivered all over.

They lay in each other's arms for a long time as they always did marveling at how they still loved and desired one another. If anything they were more in love than ever and the lovemaking was better than ever. There was not an ounce of fat on either of them and no sagging skin or bulges. Their bodies were that of persons half their ages.

They had been home six months or so when Jacob was informed there were a couple of crates from Paris at the station. He knew what was in them but he had never let on to anyone.

After he had picked the crates up and returned home Jacob had asked the family to come to dinner, telling Abby so she would have time to cook enough for everyone. The daughter's in law came to help Abby asking what Jacob was being so excited about.

"I don't have a clue!" Abby said.

The two crates were set in the parlor still nailed shut. Everyone wondered but no one asked about them. Jacob took a crow bar and removed the lid on the larger of the two crates carefully lifting out a framed painting of Abby. He looked at it before he turned it toward the rest of the family. It was beautiful! It looked just like Abby. Everyone gasped and kept saying how wonderfully the artist had caught the very essence of Abby. "This Lizzet must be a very famous painter."

Slowly Jacob removed the next item from the second box. It was wrapped in several layers of packing material. Carefully Jacob sat the object of about eighteen inches high on the table next to the fireplace.

"Oh my goodness!!" Abby cried as she went closer to examine the statuette. It was an exact replica of Weld's sculpture. It looked just as the life sized one did.

"Let me see! Let me see!" Everyone was saying. "It's so beautiful. It looks just like Weld."

Abby was holding the statuette and crying "Oh Jacob! How did you arrange this? I never saw you talking to Lizzet."

"I talked ta her that last day for about thirty minutes and swore her ta silence."

"This is the very best present you could have given me and the portrait of me is wonderful as well.

"Ho, Ho. That is mine. I'm hanging it over the fireplace so I can see it every day," Jacob informed her.

"How could Lizzet make this without Weld being present?" Everyone wanted to know.

"Lizzet still had all the measurements and sketches of Weld and she could go view the original if need be. She is very talented. To get Mama's coloring she painted a foot square with the tints of her skin. She had four squares marked off on the big square. The skin tones are different on the forehead, around the eyes and the chin and throat area."

It was time for everyone to go home. “Mornings come mighty early!” they said.

All in all, it had been a great day.

****

CHAPTER 20

A big Irishman with a quick grin came to the Bar-X-Z looking for work saying, "I ain't never worked on a ranch but I can ride purdy good, I can rope a stump and I can milk cows. We had one at home so I learned when I was a pup. I can fix a fence, clean stalls and curry down the animals. I ain't never herded a cow or branded anything. I'm a fair horseshoe player and I don't cheat at cards. I don't drink more than a couple a drinks at a settin'. Oh and I'm also a purdy durned good cook." Sean told them. "Did I tell ya, I can butcher and I can tan hides?" Sean added.

Both Weld and Bob listened to this tale winking at one another. They were remembering when they first started looking for work and listing all the things they could do.

"Where have ya worked before?" Weld asked.

"I've worked my way from New York state ta here, doin' a lot of different things. I worked digging ditches, shoveling coal, fixing up houses fer folks and drivin' folk around town to gather up supplies.

I've played fiddle and harp fer dances and I cooked fer a railroad gang. I guess ya could call me a jack of all trades."

"Are ya lookin' fer full time work or just a lay over fer awhile?" Bob asked.

"I don't guess I'm lookin' fer a forever job at ranchin' but I'll make ya a good hand while I'm around and I'll let ya know iffn I'm about ready ta leave," he stated.

"Come on over ta the bunkhouse and meet the hands. They are a good bunch of men," Weld invited.

Weld introduced Sean to the boys and soon they were swapping stories with each other.

Weld had instructed Jake to inform Sean of where to bunk and what time to show up for meals in the kitchen of the house. "Take him out tomorrow and line him out on the north side of the cow pasture fixin' fences," Weld said.

Sean was a happy Irisher. He sang, danced and played his fiddle, encouraging everyone to join in. He sang songs from his homeland in Dublin, Ireland.

Sean seemed to never tire. He worked all day and could play all night. He made trips into San Francisco to dally with the ladies. How he loved the ladies. He serenaded them with lively tunes and with ballads of love found and lost. With a lass on each arm he danced the jig then disappeared up the stairs with the both of them for a night's frolic.

Weld had pretty much traded places with Bob nowadays. Weld went into the city doing good deeds and Bob ran the ranch keeping everything running smoothly except on the weekends. Those days Bob visited Julie. They went for long rides in the country and took in theaters and civic affairs. Bob was seriously interested in Julie which fit into Weld's hopes for the future.

Fall roundup was about ready and Weld hoped Bob and the hands would agree to take on the running of the ranch and give him a few months off. He hadn't decided just where he was going but soon he would settle on the place he felt the deepest yen for. Maybe he would just travel America. There were new places and things to see right here. Maybe he would go through Arizona, over to Santa Fe, down through Texas and into Louisiana, back up through Oklahoma and into Kansas to see the folks and maybe back across Oklahoma and up into Utah. Maybe he would only cover half that area, depending on transportation and time allowing.

Tonight Weld would see Dottie for the last time before he left after approaching Bob, Jake and Slade.

Weld had spoken to Gladys last week telling her he might be gone four or more months and Bob was just as good as he at running the ranch including the bookwork. He had just done the quarterly taking care of the bank and the lawyer who had also been informed Bob would be in control while he was gone. Bob would be able to sign checks, deposit and withdraw funds for the ranch and the payroll for the hands including for him self.

When everyone was seated around the supper table, Weld broached the idea to Bob. "What do you think of me taking some time off to see a bit of our country and stopping off at the folks for a week or so?" Weld inquired.

"What do ya mean, take off?" Bob asked. "Who's gonna take care of things here?"

“Bob, ya know all about this ranch and how it is run. “Ya can do it as well as I.”

“Maybe I could and maybe I can’t. But that doesn’t mean I am.”

“Why not?” Weld asked.

“Just because I may have plans of my own.”

“If you mean that Marshall’s job, that won’t be available fer six months. I looked into it last week.” Weld informed him.

“Weld, ya son of a gun! Ya have planned this ever since I got here, haven’t ya?”

“Yep I have. Why else do ya suppose I’d be showin’ ya and tellin’ ever little detail?” Weld laughed.

“Well, since yer goin’ ta see all the folks I’ll do my best but remember, it’s a one time deal. Don’t go lookin’ ta me ever time ya get a wild hair ta travel again.”

“Ya know there is the telegraph wire and telephones in lots of places now. Maybe ya ought ta talk ta Gladys about lookin’ into the telephone thing. That way we could keep in touch better.” Weld suggested.

"It's 1913 and we have a lot of stuff available ta us now. Travel time takes about a third of the time it used ta just three or four years ago. I'm not even takin' Spike. I figure I can rent a horse or an automobile and drive most places. It's hard on a horse hauling them in a box car where it's not favorable ta ride um."

Weld packed one change of work clothes and two changes of dress clothes a dozen pair of socks as well as three sets of undergarments. He also had six neckerchiefs, one heavy coat and a light dress coat, some soap, towels and an assortment of salves for blistered feet or cracked hands. He didn't know where he might find work or what kind this time but he did not forget work gloves or his three bladed pocket knife.

Dottie cried and clung to Weld. "How can I live without your visits? You are the only person I can talk to and be myself and what about our twice a week loving time?

I really need that Weld!"

"It won't be forever little one. When I get back, we can make up fer lost time. I promise!

Their lovemaking went on all night. She just couldn't let him go. He knew every little place she needed to be loved or kissed. As always he made her feel things she had never felt with anyone else.

Weld left Dottie's just before dawn. He hated to go but the urge to see different places was just too strong. He had to go!

Weld had decided to go straight across from San Francisco, through the lower part of Nevada, into Utah where he hoped to spend a week. He would then go down into Arizona and across to New Mexico. He wanted to visit that old church and the Pueblo Indian cliff dwellings, also Santa Fe and all the museums.

He hoped to get to know some of the Indian people and hear some of their stories, if they had become civilized enough to trust the whites or if not trust them, at least not warring with them. From New Mexico, he would cross the north end of Oklahoma into Kansas to visit everyone. Afterwards he would come back through Colorado along the borders of New Mexico and Arizona, stopping in Los Angeles just to see what it was like.

He would then go back up the coast of California to San Francisco, stopping where ever there were things of interest to see or do.

He boarded the train at nine a.m. When they got underway he introduced himself to several of the people on board.

Three men in rough work clothes sat across from Weld.

"Where ya bound fer?" Weld asked.

"Utah, to the mines," one fellow offered.

"What kind of mining?" Weld wanted to know.

"Silver, right now," the same man answered.

"What does a man have ta know ta get a job mining?" Weld asked.

"Not much, except bein' willin' to work long hours for little pay and you can't be bothered by the closeness or the dark. I've seen some fellers lose control and be carried out," the smaller man explained.

"My name is Weld Winter. What's yours?"

The big fellow said, "My name is Jason, this skinny one is Tim."

"And I'm John," piped up the freckled faced man.

"How about introducing me to whoever does the hiring?" Weld implored.

"Sure, come along, but I don't know why a feller like you would want to grub in a dirty mine."

The mine was about two miles from the small mining town. The houses were small unpainted dreary affairs. Small children and dogs ran and played. The children's clothes were patched and either too large or too small. The women he saw were unhappy looking, unsmiling. There didn't seem to be many elderly folks around. The three men who accompanied Weld told him, "Folks don't live to be of old age mining."

The first time Weld went down into a mine he got a real sinking feeling. It felt as though he had been going down for hours. When he stepped off the caged platform he had trouble walking. He tried to stay close to Jason or one of the other boys but the head- man put him on the other side and up further ahead explaining what to do and also how to listen for shuddering timbers or scaling rock. Jason was right. It was hard work but he enjoyed it, humming softly to himself. He was glad the work at the ranch had kept his hands calloused and tough otherwise swinging that pick would have had his hands bleeding in the first hour.

He was shown a rock formation with silver ore so he could recognize it if he saw it again. When the whistle blew to change shifts he was ready. "This is hard work," he thought but he would be back tomorrow.

Jason invited Weld to bunk with him, Tim and John. Weld whistled and sang as he bathed and changed clothes.

"What is there to do around here after work?" Weld asked.

"Not much hereabouts. We have to go into Ogden or Salt Lake if we want to find much goin's on," John said.

"Don't ya have a place here fer people ta git together? Ya know, ta have music and dancin' and the like?"

"Well, there is an empty building and some boxes for chairs. An old wobbly table serves as a game table when some of the boys get together to play some cards."

"How about the women folk and the younguns? Where do they go ta relax?" Weld asked.

"I guess they ain't no place for that sorta thing," John said.

"Can ya walk me down ta this buildin' ya are talkin' about."

"Sure! But as I told ya it's just an old abandoned building," Jim offered.

Weld whistled through his teeth and hummed as he walked around the room. It was about 30x30 feet with an old fireplace on the north side. It looked like with a good chimney cleaning and replacing a couple of stones it would work fine.

"Can we find someone to work on cleaning the place and on putting some paint on the inside? Where can I buy some chairs and a couple of tables? The ladies will need a place ta put patterns and sewing supplies while they visit with neighbors and while the children play together. Do any of the folks ya know have any instruments, or play one, or sing?" Weld wanted to know.

"Just what is it you are figuring on?" John asked.

"I noticed as we came into camp the children and the womenfolk seem ta be unhappy. The little ones don't seem ta have any place ta play except the road. I think if we put our minds ta it, we could make a difference in a good way, a way for people ta get interested and involved instead of just sitting or standing gazing at the emptiness. What day do we have off?" Weld wanted to know.

"When we have a full crew we can get off week ends, if not we have to stay and cover."

"How about now? Do we have full crews?"

"Yep, we do," John informed Weld.

"Does any one have a rig ta carry furniture and lumber?"

"I have a wagon but no hoss," Tim said.

"Well my brother has a team of horses he would loan me," Jason offered.

"Fine!" Weld laughed. "We will go when we get off duty Friday. In the meantime let's find some help ta start the cleanup work," Weld advised.

Weld hired three women to do the cleanup and someone had donated paint and brushes. One husband fixed the stones in the fireplace and nailed all the loose boards in the floors and the walls. He fixed the sagging door as well.

Weld bought lumber to make benches for plank tables. He also bought four rocking chairs, not new but solid.

There was a bolt of blue material for curtains. A small cot was installed for babies to be put down for their naps.

Weld bought toys for both girls and boys. He also bought rope for lassos.

"My, my! How this place has changed!" everyone marveled.

Weld had found half dozen people with fiddles, harps, banjos and juice harps. The next weekend, Weld had gathered singers, dancers, musicians and jugglers. He could hardly believe there were two jugglers in this small community. Everyone had a great time. Weld sang, did a jig and did rope tricks. He danced with the ladies whose husbands allowed them to dance. There were no unmarried ladies. It seemed as soon as a girl came of age they fled to greener pastures so to speak.

People's faces were alive and happy looking. The children laughed happily as they played with their new toys. Weld used twenty feet of the rope to make a swing for the children. He told them to take turns and for the larger children to be careful with the smaller ones.

Weld moved on into Arizona, leaving good friends and good feelings behind. He also liked feeling as though he had helped someone and had left part of himself behind in the memories of good people.

Weld arrived just in time to rent a horse for a few days. He picked a broad chested spirited horse with three white stockings that put him in mind of Spike. He tied a new bedroll, with his belongings and a frying pan, jerky and hard tack along with an oversized canteen.

Weld rode into the cliff dweller's ruins, keeping an eye out for disgruntled Indians. He just had to see the ruins up close if possible. He hoped he could meet a friendly Indian, who could tell him about the history of the place, the pre-historic times. He wanted to see that lake that everybody told him about.

Weld was whistling softly as he rode but he heard the rider picking his way through the rocks and sand. When he turned Weld, was confronted by an Indian brave of about his own age. The brave sat his pony with ease.

Weld raised his right hand in a gesture of friendship. The Indian sat stoically not blinking an eye. Weld offered the brave some water from his canteen. The brave took it, drank lightly and returned the canteen to Weld.

"Do ya speak English? How about Spanish? Como te llamas?"

The brave replied in broken English. "What you want here?"

"To see the cliff dwellings and find out the history of the cliff dwellers just for my own experience," Weld answered.

"My people say there was a great drought lasted for thirty some years hundreds years past. The people abandoned the cliff cities. Their descendants were living in fortified towns near watercourses at the time some Spanish expedition came about five hundred years ago, so my people believe. Come, I will take you to the ropes that will get you into some of the cliff caves."

The Indian headed toward the south end of a row of cliff openings. There he stood on his horse parted some bushes and pulled down a knotted rope. He hauled himself hand over hand to the first opening and dropped the rope back down to Weld.

Weld was enthralled with imaginings of what it was like back then. He could visualize families happy and laughing, caring for each other.

Zeume told Weld he would take him to see his father further on up past the cliff caves. Weld accepted gladly.

As they rode into the Indian camp many angry eyed people walked toward them. Zueme held his hand up, saying something Weld could not understand. Most of the expressions changed and became friendly looking except for two young braves standing by the wigwam of the chief.

Zueme spoke to his father in English saying, "This man comes in peace to learn of our people the cliff dwellers. He has a pure heart. I have told him that you can tell him of the cliff people and of pre-historic times here on our reservation." The chief invited Weld to share their food and to stay the night.

The next day Zueme and his father told Weld of the past history as it was handed down to the present time. Weld was very happy with his luck at finding Zueme and his people.

He spent two more days just riding and enjoying the outdoors seeing everything.

Weld next went to Santa Fe, New Mexico. New Mexico had just been admitted to statehood a year before. The Pueblo Indians also had cliff dwellers. They still had spiraling cliff like abodes.

He visited the museums and the Mission Church with the thick walls where the Indians as well as everyone else visited. The buildings were of adobe, cool in the summer and warm in the winter.

The driver he employed knew every point of interest and took him to every one of them. Weld spent six days in Santa Fe before he got on his way to Albuquerque, New Mexico. There he visited some in Old Town where Indians and Whites sold silver, turquoise and Navajo blankets.

Weld found a woman that made the best Mexican food he had ever tasted. A steady stream of hungry men came to eat Rosa's food. Here Weld became friendly with many of the area's people. There was much anger and mistrust of the white race but as usual Weld was able to gain the trust of those he came into contact with.

He joined their dances and enjoyed entertaining them with his harmonica and borrowed ropes to do his twirling, dancing a jig as he twirled the large circle of rope. He knew one song in Spanish. His accent was pretty good too.

Weld crossed into the Oklahoma panhandle and on up into Kansas and on to his family's farm. He entered the house quietly and sat down in his father's large leather chair in front of the fireplace. In about thirty minutes Mama would be coming down to start breakfast so he got up and started the fire in the great kitchen stove got the coffee pot filled and placed on one of the front lids of the stove. He would wait for his mother to add the coffee. She did it so much better than the rest of the family. Weld wasn't a coffee drinker but most of the family was.

He heard Abby on the stairs. He sat quietly at the kitchen table. At first Abby did not see him but noticed the fire made and the coffee pot on the stove.

She turned toward the door she had just entered and nearly collapsed not expecting anyone to be up.

"Oh my goodness Weld, it's you. When did you get here? Why didn't you let us know?" she rambled as she squeezed him. "Jacob! Come here! Hurry! Hurry!" she called out.

Jacob was still buttoning his shirt as he entered the kitchen.

"Weld! Son! Come here," as he grabbed Weld and hugged him and patted his back asking questions a mile a minute.

"Where are the boys?" Weld asked.

"Oh that's right, you don't know. We have a little different set up now. The married boys only work three days a week they have their own farms to take care of. Henry is still full time but is off on weekends as well as Jack. Everyone is paid by the hour now. We have two part time hands that are working out pretty good and we sold all the milk cows except two. We now have a fine herd of beef cattle which don't take up nearly the time milk cows do. We've added extra chickens and sell fryers all year round. The extra hens give us extra eggs ta sell so income is about the same," Jacob stated.

"Sounds like ya have made a good change but where's Henry and Jack now?"

"They will be makin' an entrance any time now. Ya know how young fellers tom cat. Well they are no different so the stay abed until the last moment."

About that second both men walked into the kitchen grinning and punching each other on the shoulders. Noticing Weld both of them grabbed onto him shaking his hand and nudging him. "Glad ta see ya," they both said.

“Man both of ya have grown a heap and ya are lookin’ good,” Weld told them.

Abby was busily making breakfast loving to see her boys together. Today all of them would be there together except for Bob. She wished he and Jenny could be there as well. She did so dread seeing them all grown and leaving home. Oh she wanted them to have their own lives, loves and families she just felt so useless with them gone. Of course there was still the three younguns that would be at home for several years yet.

The two new hands arrived for breakfast just as Abby called for everyone to sit down. Weld was introduced and the talk fest continued.

The young girls never breakfasted with the grownups because usually that was the time work was laid out and they had business discussions. Also it was too early for children.

Jack and Henry got up took their hats off the rack and started for the barn followed by the two new hands.

“I’ll be down ta where ya are workin’ today after I visit with Mama and Papa. I’d like ta see the girls too. I’ve brought them some presents from the Indian people in Santa Fe, New Mexico and for Mama as well," Weld told them.

Weld filled Jacob and Abby in on the ranch and Bob. "He is a very good rancher he can run the physical part of the ranch work and now he has learned about the business end of ranching, handling men and everything in between."

"Bob, I think is pretty much gone on a fine lady in San Francisco and I believe she feels the same. She is a blueblood, wealthy, beautiful and does so much good for people less fortunate than she. Ya spent time with her in San Francisco when ya were workin' the soup kitchens didn't ya Mama?" Weld asked.

"I met Julie. She is a wonderful young woman."

"Bob has his mind set on continuing ta work as a Marshall but I believe he will one day go into Government law. Maybe the legislative branch or head up some charitable concern. He has been working hard ta find help fer so many. He finds jobs fer men and has set up area childcare so the mothers can try ta find work of some kind. He is teachin' a class on sums, ta a group of boys fourteen, sixteen and up. Gladys teaches the six years old and up, readin', spellin' and writin'. She enjoys workin' with the children."

"Gladys hasn't heard anything from her daughter in London since she got home. when Jenny writes ta me and says anything about Gilly, I always let Gladys know. She pretends she isn't interested but she is. She worries about Gilly like any mother would."

Jacob was eager to show Weld his 'Tin Lizzy' he had purchased just last month. "She's a beauty!" Jacob bragged. "It takes no time at all ta go into town and back. Ya can't get her stuck in the mud. She has those tall wheels that keep her high off the ground. She goes almost forty miles an hour, course I don't drive half that. It doesn't take a load of tools ta keep her runnin' like those other automobiles. Abby drives ta town alone ta get supplies fer the kitchen and goes to visit the girls and the wives of the boys. She really enjoys the thing."

Mildred, Harriet and Rosie came down for breakfast. Seeing Weld they squealed and rushed into his arms.

"My goodness!! How all of ya have grown. I was expectin' three small children."

"Brother it's been over three years since you saw us so naturally we have grown," Mildred said.

Weld got out his carpetbag and brought out Indian dolls with colorful Indian dresses and long braids. He also had three silver and turquoise bracelets for the girls. Weld handed his mother a silver and turquoise squash blossom necklace.

"Oh how beautiful!" Abby cried. "This is so pretty. Thank you so much son, I shall cherish it always."

For Jacob and all the boys he had handmade leather belts with turquoise insets on silver buckles. For Raye he had a wide silver bracelet with turquoise inlay. For his three sister's in law, he had tortoise shell combs for their hair with turquoise across the top of each comb.

There was much oooing and ahhhing over the presents from those in the kitchen. The rest of the presents would have to wait for the rest of the family to arrive at the farm.

"Come in here son," Jacob said. "I have somethin' ta show ya."

Jacob opened the curtains and lit a lamp. Standing in front of the fireplace he pointed to the portrait of Abby. “Mama! How beautiful ya are but how did ya git it done and brought here?” Weld asked.

“Just the same way we got this,” she said, pointing to the statuette of Weld.

“My goodness! How on earth did ya git that? I didn’t sit for a small one” he said.

“No but Lizzet still had the sketches and measurements. She just made this and shipped it to us. Isn’t it the most beautiful thing in the world?” Abby declared.

“Uhh, I guess it’s a good piece of artwork,” Weld admitted. “Lizzet is a great artist, whether painting or sculpting. Just look how she captured your inner beauty as well as your outer beauty,” Weld said.

Abby said, “I was very surprised when these things arrived. I had never seen Jacob talking to Lizzet.”

“I spent about half an hour with Lizzet. I’m pretty slick,” Jacob laughed. “She assured me she could finish both the portrait and the statue and ship them here.”

"We had a wonderful trip but once in a lifetime is enough for me. If we do any more traveling it will be here in America," Jacob told them.

Weld said, "I guess I'll see if I can't find the boys and give them a hand. What time will Jerry and the others be here?"

"Umm, let me think. Is it a workday for them today? Yes, Carl and Frank will be showing up here any minute now. Jerry works tomorrow," Jacob informed him. "We can drive around and see all of them later today," Jacob assured weld. "We can make arrangements for a whing ding for this Saturday."

"Sounds good ta me," Weld laughed. "Nothin' I like better than a real get together with family and friends."

Abby was listening thinking of how many pretty young girls she could invite, knowing Weld's affinity for the ladies. Many a girl had set the caps for Weld but none of them had really caught his eye.

He never played favorites. He flirted danced and complimented each of them the same. Weld had such a loving, caring side to him for all humanity, it just bubbled out of him. Abby thought, "I don't believe I've ever heard a single person speak unkindly of Weld, even while he was growing up."

When the rest of the boys tangled up Weld was the peacemaker. Of all of Abby's children, Weld was her favorite. Not that she loved him any more than the rest, he was just the most giving, loving and helpful not only toward his own family but to everyone he met.

Abby looked out the window and watched Weld driving the 'Tin Lizzy' all over the yard and the barnyard as well. He and Jacob were laughing enjoying just being together. They drove out the gate heading for the road going to the other boy's homes she bet. All of them would be here for supper, so she began preparing for them. Abby hadn't felt so good since before the two girls and three boys left home to marry.

Jacob and Weld drove into Jerry's yard about ten a.m. Carly came out to greet them. Seeing Weld, she ran and hugged him. "It's so good to see you!" she said. Jerry will be so happy to see you."

"Where is Jerry?" Jacob asked.

"He is mending harnesses in the tack room I believe," she informed them.

Jacob and Weld headed for the barn. Sure enough Jerry was working on a harness that had lost its trace line ring. He hadn't seen or heard his father or brother come in.

"Hey!" Weld said loudly. "Do I have a brother around here name of Jerry?"

Jerry dropped his harness and rose to meet Weld and his father.

"I know ya will never believe this but I was just sittin' here thinkin' how much I would love ta see ya. It's been three years or more since ya been home. Man ya are a sight fer sore eyes. Have ya seen Carl or Frank yet? Ya must have seen Jack and Henry and the younguns."

So far Weld couldn't get a word in to answer. "Come up ta the house fer somethin' ta drink and ta visit a spell," Jerry urged.

"Not now," Jacob said. "We have ta drive ta see the rest of the family and git back fer supper that I'm sure Abby is preparing fer everybody tonight. We are having a real whing ding Saturday so everyone free up that day and night and be there today by suppertime. Ya might send Carly ta help your mother with the fixin's tonight.

Weld just smiled and agreed to whatever anyone said. He still hadn't had a chance to speak but finally got in "I brought all of ya a little gift. I'll give um ta ya tonight when we are all together," he promised. "Married life must agree with ya cause ya look real good," Weld added.

Jacob left word with the boy's wives and with his daughter to be at the house for supper tonight. Not stopping for chit-chat because he thought Abby might need to go into town for supplies or something and would need the 'Tin Lizzy.'

When they got back to the ranch, Abby was ready to bite nails. She did have to go or send someone to pick up special fixings for supper. She pleaded for Jacob and Weld to go so she could continue to pluck chickens getting them ready to fry for supper. She also had to make some pies and a big chocolate cake.

Jacob told her the girls would be there in about an hour so not to get in a hurry. "There is plenty of time but we will git your fixin's if ya write em down."

Weld walked over and hugged Abby to his chest. "I've missed all of ya so much." He said, "I love ya Mama."

Abby had tears in her eyes. “He is so sweet,” she thought.

The girls had come and each had brought a favorite dish. They all went right to work telling Abby to rest a while. She did!

Everyone talked at once discussing Weld’s surprise visit and how wonderful he looked. He had promised them all presents. What could he have brought? Maybe a book, or candy, they guessed. “Mama, do you know what he has for us?”

“No I cannot say I do. You will just have to wait until he is ready to give them to you.”

“Now does that mean she doesn’t know or won’t say?” they giggled.

Weld and Jacob arrived with Abby’s order. The girls all pounced on Weld. “What did you bring us?” they demanded.

“Oh that will have ta wait until everyone is here,” he said laughing.

“Oh no! That’s not fair. Tell us now,” they begged.

Weld just turned his palms up in an, I can’t help it gesture and went out the door with his father.

Weld thought his father had laughed more in this one day than he had ever seen him laugh in any other day he could remember. Life seemed perfect for his parents he thought. The farm was much easier to run now they had no money worries and they were still deeply in love with one another. "How wonderful!" Weld marveled.

Weld would find out what girls were still single from Henry and Jackson tonight. He knew or had known a bevy of young ladies before he had left home but he knew that many of them would be married or gone by now. There was no special girl. He still had no interest in marriage but he was very interested in good times dancing, kissing and romancing, just as long as they knew it was just playtime for him. He could hardly wait for Saturday.

About five thirty every family member began showing up hugging Weld and shaking his hand.

"Where ya been? Whatcha been doin? Are ya back ta stay?" the questions came fast and furious.

"I have ta be back at the Bar-X-Z before 1914. Bob gave me these four months off and I've used up a third of that all ready. I've been to

Utah, Arizona, New Mexico, Oklahoma and here. I stopped in a mining community, worked in a mine and helped build a small community clubhouse. I traveled around Arizona meeting the Indian people and visiting cliff dwellings where hundreds of years ago people lived, raised families and were happy. I spent many days in around Santa Fe where many of the Pueblo Indians still live in sort of stacked adobe buildings. They join the white traders in selling pottery, blankets and the like. I then went to Albuquerque and stayed in Old Town, joining in on their dances, music and Indian turquoise and silver Indian jewelry making."

"Speaking of Indian handy work, I brought each of you a small gift I hope ya will like," Weld said as he opened his carpetbag removing belts for all the boys and Jacob.

"Dang boys! Ain't these great!" Carl said. Everyone agreed.

Next he handed Raye the wide silver bracelet with the large turquoise center. Raye hugged Weld saying, "Thank you brother! I love it."

Next came the beautiful tortoise shell combs for the girl's hair sporting turquoise insets. "Oh how beautiful!" the girls gasped. "I've never seen anything like this before." Each girl embarrassed Weld thanking him for his thoughtfulness.

The three little girls came in showing off their bracelets and dolls to everyone. Abby undid the buttons at the neck of her dress displaying the lovely squash blossom necklace. It was laden with turquoise all down both sides and the largest turquoise setting of them all in the center where it dipped between Abby's cleavage.

"Beautiful! Beautiful!" They exclaimed. "How wonderful and savages make these?" they asked.

"Not savages, people. People just like you and me. They love, they cry, they bleed when cut and they have feelings just like we do. They are wonderful people," Weld stated. "I feel honored ta have spent time with them."

Jacob brought out the instruments and Raye sat at the piano. Each boy took up their favorite instrument and everyone sang, mostly hymns. Weld insisted on Danny Boy, of which he sang lead. He offered to teach them to do the Irish Jig but only the little girls would try. Everyone laughed and clapped for the children.

"We all have ta work tomorrow bright and early and it's almost nine p.m. We must go," everyone agreed. "Saturday we can play all day and all night if we want to. Thanks so much for the presents. We love ya."

"Thank ya all for coming, it's been great," Weld admitted. "I'll see all of ya everday while I'm here or as much as I can anyway."

The girls had cleaned the kitchen, taking leftovers with them to feed their husbands on the morrow.

All the boys and Raye too seem to be very content with their lives," Weld opined.

"Yes I believe they are happy," Abby said, "I haven't heard any complaints from either side."

"Ya know, I'm ready ta hit the hay if it's all right with ya," Weld told his parents.

"Sure son. We are going to bed as well. Your old room is ready for you," Abby said.

Weld's head had barely hit the pillow before he was fast asleep. He dreamed of Dottie, of making love to her, of holding her in his arms. Blissfully he slept.

The morning brought all the brothers together except Bob, for a day's work on the farm. Weld opted to ride fence with Carl the first half day. They talked as they rode of growing up and the wonderful times they had always enjoyed. Carl spoke of his wife and marriage in general. He was very happy and they planned to start a family very soon.

Weld discussed Bar-X-Z in detail and his role there and how Bob fitted in right from the first. "Bob likes the outdoors. That was part of why he became a Marshall," Weld said. "Ya know? Bob doesn't sow many wild oats. He has this thing about right and wrong and says the door swings both ways. If it is not acceptable for ladies ta be loose then it's not all right fer men either," Weld informed Carl.

That afternoon Weld hooked up with Henry and Jack to clean up the barn stalls and fork hay into the animals. They laughingly handed Weld the shovel to scoop manure. "This shovel just don't fit my hand," Jack told Weld.

"Give me the rundown on the unmarried gals still available and who I should stay away from," Weld said.

"How about Nancy Shear? Is she still around or Elsie Woods? Now that is one pretty doll," Weld remembered.

Both boys laughed. You wouldn't know her now. She has three younguns and has gained at least fifty pounds. We will take ya around Friday night so ya look over the field," Henry said.

"Ya know me. I want no one who wants ta be serious. I'm just here fer a few days and I ain't ready ta settle on any one girl just yet," Weld swore.

"Yeah we know. There are still too many women needing ta hear soft words and tender touches from Weld, the great lover."

"No, that ain't it. I need the tender touches and I need to feel needed. The ladies never cease ta show how caring they are. Women want ta be loved just like we do," Weld explained. I just love ta take time ta let them know how beautiful they are."

"I'll tell ya this, there is a lot of them that still ask about ya," Jack offered.

At the supper table the boys had a good laugh telling how Weld did such a good job cleaning the stables.

"Oh you ornery boys. Weld you don't have to clean stables," Abby scolded.

"I don't mind in the least. It all has ta be done," Weld opined.

"Now don't you boys go putting off the nastiest chores onto Weld just because he is so easy going," Abby said.

Jacob spoke up, "Don't ya worry 'bout Weld. No one forces him ta do anything he doesn't want ta do."

Weld just grinned.

"I think I'll go into town and look around," Weld said. I want ta look up some old friends and maybe play some cards."

"Yeah cards!" Henry grinned.

Jacob insisted that Weld take the Tin Lizzy. "It's faster and easier."

Nothing had drastically changed. There were just a lot more horseless carriages a new false front over the hotel where he usually stayed while in town and a new eating place called Sally's. A big tall tree had been taken out from in front of the blacksmith's place. The large sign over Neil's Saloon, had been replaced by a sign saying

Mary's Place. Weld could hear music and laughter coming from Mary's Place and decided to investigate.

The bar had been lengthened about six feet. A small stage was next to the piano and all the tables were set up to accommodate four persons, except for three of them which would serve only two. There were several men and two women customers seated facing the stage. Women in a saloon was new to Weld, except for the working girls of course.

Weld stepped up to the bar ordered a drink and asked, "Where's Mary?"

"She don't come down 'til showtime," the fat bartender said.

"When is that?" Weld inquired.

"'Bout seven today," the fat man said. "She don't fool round here except whenever she sings."

Weld decided to stay until this Mary came down. Maybe there was something special about this woman.

"How long has this place been Mary's Place?" Weld inquired.

"Umm, 'bout six months, I guess."

"How's business since a woman owns it?" Weld wanted to know.

"Better than it was before, quiet a bit better," he was told.

At about fifteen before seven lamps were lit on stage with reflectors on the sides next to the audience shining the light on whoever was on stage. Most of the lamps were turned down or off in the rest of the building. When the music started to play a beautiful woman in a fitted off the shoulder silk gown appeared as if by magic on the stage, swaying to the music in a graceful motion. Her hair was jet black, long lashes and light stage makeup, enough to look lovely but not the thick harsh makeup most performers used. Her dress shimmered and glowed on her perfect body and when she began to sing, not a word escaped anyone in the audience. They were all spellbound, including Weld.

He had been to many of the great theaters abroad but none could compare with this Mary.

Weld sent a note backstage asking Mary to please grant him an audience saying, "My name is Weld Winter. I'm in town visiting my family for a short time. Would you consider having a late supper with me?"

Mary's maid always went through the requests from people wanting to see her, only allowing Mary to see those that seemed gentlemanly and this one seemed to be the only one in that class this evening. She lay the note on Mary's make up vanity waiting for an answer one way or the other.

Mary nodded yes and Vera went to find Mr. Winter. Vera ushered Weld into Mary's dressing room and closed the door behind her on the way out. She would be near enough to answer Mary's call for help if she needed it and her little derringer was in the pocket of her smock.

Weld walked the five steps it took to lift Mary's delicate hand to his lips, where he placed a light kiss upon it. "I am so glad you would see me," Weld admitted. "You are the most beautiful and talented lady I have ever had the pleasure of meeting."

"Thank you sir!" Mary said. "I was impressed with your manners contained in your note. For the most part invitations that I receive are not so elegant," she smiled.

"Where would you prefer to dine?" Weld asked.

"It really makes little difference to me. I eat very little these days," she informed him.

"When ya eat, what kind of food do ya prefer?" Weld probed.

"Just plain fare."

"I know of a little place that serves Chinese Duck with almonds, a mixed salad and Won Ton soup," Weld baited her.

"That sounds wonderful!"

Weld helped her on with her wrap and took her arm guiding her through the side entrance of the building.

"How thoughtful of him," Mary thought. "Most others would have wanted to push through the crowd just to prove he was able to win a date with Mary."

The small place he took her to was dimly lit and quiet. No one stared or bothered them as they talked and ate the delicious food.

Mary told Weld this was the very nicest thing that had happened to her since her child and husband had been killed by a horse drawn carriage runaway. They could not get out of the way of the frightened animals. Her baby had died instantly her husband two days later.

Weld was solicitous, holding her hand gently. "That is so terrible. How hard it must be for you to be on stage singing of happy things while your heart breaks. I am so sorry."

"No, it really helps me. I love performing and lose myself in the moment."

"That is so fortunate fer ya."

****

CHAPTER 21

Henry was standing by Jacob's Tin Lizzy when Weld and Mary came out of the restaurant. Henry was looking worriedly at Weld. He took off his hat, looking at Mary. "I'm sorry ta intrude maam," he said, "but I'm Weld's brother and there has been an accident at home. Weld, Dad has been kicked by that new stallion he bought, it's bad."

Weld turned to Mary. "Please get in Miss. I'll take ya home then I have ta be goin' ta my father and Mama.

"Of course Mr. Winter. I'm so sorry. Just let me off in front I'll be all right."

"No ma'am, I'll see ya safely in," Weld insisted. "May I call on ya when Papa is better?"

"Yes, please do and let me know how your father is."

The doctor's rig was at the farm and so were all the boys and their wives. Raye and her husband were there also. Weld felt a terrible weight pressing him down. "Please God, don't take my Dad. We all need him so much."

When he entered the house he knew it was over. Everyone was crying and hugging each other. They looked as though they would never smile again.

Abby was sitting at the kitchen table her head bowed, no tears. She had a look of utter despair as if she had lost her whole life. Weld kneeled beside her touching her face, kissing her hands. "Mama, Mama, we all love ya, we need ya. We need your strength. Let us help ya as ya have always helped us. Papa will always be with us now. He'll be watchin' over us forever. We boys will take care of everything. Don't worry."

Abby reached over and smoothed Weld's hair saying, "Yes son, we will be fine but right now I need to lie down. I just feel all poured out." Weld took his mother's arm and guided her into his room. Papa still lay in their bed. He closed the door quietly putting his index finger to his lips, asking everyone to be as quiet as possible.

They all sat around the kitchen table where they had sat for so many years with Jacob at the head of the table. From there he had given instructions for the day's chores and appointing which chore was to be done and by whom. How could they ever survive without him? Who could they find answers from when in doubt about a crop or an animal or any problem they might have. Jacob had always been there with the right word, the right way. The whole family depended on him.

The family members with animals to take care of returned to their homes. That left only Weld, Henry, Jack the three young children and Abby.

No one slept much. They were very tired but could not sleep.

Weld worried over his mother. She looked so exhausted and sad. How was he going to break this to Bob? It was much too far away for him to have any hopes of coming here. Henry and Jack had gone downtown to that telegraph place to see if there was a way to get word to Bob. Weld didn't know what they had learned. He had, had no chance to talk to them.

Weld was up before daylight making ready to cook for the hands as well as for the family. He had flapjack batter ready, bacon in a large frying pan, eggs set out waiting until time to fry. The table was set, except Jacob's place, tall glasses were out for milk with syrup, jams, jellies and butter. The coffee pot was bubbling merrily and smelled good even if he had made it himself. It might not taste good but it sure did smell great.

Henry was the first to arrive in the kitchen, followed by two of the new hands and finally Jack made an appearance looking sad and forlorn.

"Good mornin' fellers," Weld said to all of them. "How did ya all rest?"

All shook their heads no indicating no one really rested.

"Take it easy today boys. Just tend the animals. Feed and water the chickens and gather the eggs. They were not gathered yesterday. Be sure and store them on the right side wall so's not ta git the fresh mixed up with the older boxes," suggested Weld.

About that time Abby came into the kitchen. She hadn't even gotten out of her clothes from yesterday Weld noticed. "Mama, go back ta bed. I'll bring yer breakfast ta ya."

She answered by taking the flapjack turner out of his hand saying, "This is my job. I thank you for helping today but I'll be fine."

"Mama, please let me help ya. I can cook almost as good as ya and I really enjoy it. I don't git much chance at the Bar-X-Z cause we have a cook and Gladys as well" he pled.

"Maybe you can prepare supper," she said. "But I'm here now. Pour the coffee and milk and sit down. PLEASE!" she said.

The boys managed a grin. Mama was still in control. Everything was gonna work out they thought.

The hands had just left after thanking Abby and Weld for a fine breakfast, tipping their hats to her when the three little girls came in. "Do ya want flapjacks?" Weld asked them.

"Yes please, with one bacon and one egg."

"How many flapjacks, one?"

"Yes, one," they all said.

"Papa always had four and three eggs plus four strips of bacon," Harriet informed them.

As soon as everyone had been served, Abby left. She went back into Weld's room and lay down again in her same clothes. She just couldn't go into her room to get clean things. Later if some of the girls came she would send them to get her a change of everything and she would bathe. For now she would just sleep she decided.

Raye came about nine a.m. Weld had cleaned the kitchen sparkling clean. They never said a word to each other. They just hugged standing for a long time rocking back and forth.

Finally Weld said, “Go ta Mama. She’s in my room. I think she may want some help with her clothing and bath water,” he told Raye.

Mama was fast asleep on top of the covers fully dressed even with her shoes and stockings. Raye went her parent’s room keeping her eyes averted from the bed. She got Abby’s clothes and returned to where Abby slept. She did not awaken her.

Raye went into the kitchen and put large pots of water to heat for Abby’s bath. Every once in a while she would peek in on Abby, waiting for her to awaken.

When noon came and Abby still had not woken, Raye called Weld to accompany her to check on Abby. They did not try to enter quietly but Abby slept on. Weld, went to his mother touching her face and forehead and then her arms, they were cold.

"Mama! Mama!" Weld cried. "Wake up dear. Raye has brought your clean clothes and the water is hot for your bath." Abby did not wake. She was dead.

"Raye run ta the barn and bring the boys! Hurry!"

"What is it Weld? What is it?" Raye demanded.

"I don't know!" Weld lied. "Just hurry!"

Raye ran out of the house screaming for the boys.

"Come quickly! Hurry! Something's wrong with Mama!"

They came at a run following Raye to Weld's room.

Weld had placed her head on a pillow and had pulled the sheet up to her chest.

Abby looked asleep. She had a sweet little smile on her face. The same smile all of them had seen her flash to Papa hundreds of times.

This just could not be happening, both parents dead within fourteen hours of each other. Jacob had been killed by a horse but Abby had been in perfect health.

"I guess they just could not be apart. She went to him to be with him as she always had been," Weld said fighting tears and rage.

Jack went to give the bad news to Jerry, Carl and Frank.

"Oh don't tell me that!" Jerry demanded. "Ya never joke on a thing like that."

Jerry saw tears in Frank's eyes and he knew it was true. "How? When?" He wanted to know. "How could this happen? Why? Why?"

Frank just fell to his knees and pounded the ground weeping aloud. "What have we done ta deserve this? What?

"Oh Jack, what will we do? What can we do? Our entire foundation is gone."

"No it isn't Jerry. We still have each other and ya married fellers have wives ta help ya and we all have God. With our faith and our health, we will suffer but we will survive."

Jerry looked at his younger brother full of wisdom, counting their blessings. He was right. They would survive and help each other as always. "Let's go." Jerry said.

They stopped by Carl's, who agreed to have his wife pick up the rest of the family. Once again they gathered in their familiar places at the kitchen table. No one was saying much. They sat in stunned silence, hearts breaking, eyes swollen and red.

After the funeral, people went to the farm, bringing loads of cooked foods. The men went to the barn, the women gathered in the kitchen and living room. Everybody spoke in subdued voices. Everyone trying to grasp how such a thing could happen to any one, least of all people like the Winter family. There wasn't a single one of them that any one had heard anything bad gossip about. You could always turn to any or all of them to help out in any kind of difficulty most having done so at one time or another.

At the barn, everyone was turning to Weld to ask about the farm. "Who would be taking charge?"

Weld said he would get hold of Bob to see if he could stay on at the Bar-X-Z for awhile longer giving Weld time to figure what would be the best way to handle things.

No one knew if his folks had left a will or not. They would have to find out before they started anything and Weld had to find out about Bob's feelings on things.

A feller drove up to the front step holding a piece of paper looking for Weld Winter. "He's in the barn." Raye informed the man who strode toward the barn.

"Weld Winter?" The man asked, holding the piece of paper before him.

"Yes, I'm Weld Winter." Weld assured him. "Can I help ya?"

"Maybe I can help you. This here's a telegram from Californey." The man handed Weld the piece of paper asking, "Will thur be an answer? I kin take it back wid me so's yuh don't hafta go inta town yerself," he boasted.

Weld opened the telegram, reading it to the group. "So sorry to hear bad news.-stop- Take as long as you need.-stop- Give my love to all.—stop- signed Bob."

"Yes, there will be an answer." Weld told the man. "Address it ta Bob Winter in care of Bar-X-Z, San Francisco, California. More bad news.—stop- Mama died this day.—stop- send your ideas on how to handle farm. -stop- signed Weld."

Weld paid the man, feeling a little less pressure and hating the fact that Bob could not be here now.

That night they searched for a will or some kind of information saying what the folks had wanted done in connection with everything and where everything was. The little children came to say good night and asked what everyone was looking for.

"Oh just some papers about Mama and Papa's business stuff."

Harriet walked over to the window seat, moved a little latch and opened the lid to the storage space. Inside were a big envelope and two ledgers, also there were the furs that Bob had sent home. There was a deal of money and legal stuff, like marriage licenses, babies birth documents, ownership papers on the livestock, the farm, the machinery etc. "Is that what you are looking for?" Harriet asked.

"Yes it is. How did you know where it was?" Raye asked.

"Mama showed me. She said to always remember in case she forgot," she beamed.

No will was found, but a letter from the lawyer stated that the will was ready for their signature. It was dated just before they went to London. Weld thought, "They just wanted to have things in order in case the ship sank," he smiled a tiny smile.

"We have forgotten all about Jenny," Weld cried. "We must see if that telegram goes to England," he said as he headed out the door.

"Weld, ya can't do it tonight. It won't open until nine a.m. tomorrow."

"It won't? Well I'll be there ready and a waitin' when they do open," he swore, which he was.

Weld really needed to see Dottie. He needed to hold and to be held for just a little while he thought.

His mind went to Mary. Maybe he could just talk to her. That would make him feel better. Hesitating a little he knocked on Mary's side door. Vera saw who it was and had him wait until she could find out if Mary could see him just now. She came back to the door and bade him enter. He knew he looked a fright but it couldn't be helped just now. She looked lovely. Her eyes were so blue they looked like blue indigo. "Could we please sit down?" He asked. "I'm so tired I don't think I can stand another moment."

"Sit here," she offered, patting a chaise. You can rest while we talk.

He kept hold of her hand, kissing it and the tips of her fingers. He finally got out that both parents were dead not having enough strength to give details just now. He leaned over, his head touching her lap and went sound asleep. When she attempted to remove her hand, he held it tighter in his sleep. Finally she just moved a little straighter, keeping his head in her lap. She stroked his face and hair. He really was a fine looking man, she noted. He had so much heart ache right now. Eventually he would be better, but for right now he needed someone to let down to, someone to make him feel cared for.

It had been so long since she had touched or been touched by a man and she missed it. She missed the conversations and the back rubs the kissing and the lovemaking. She was a good woman. Many did not believe she was because she ran a saloon and entertained the public. The only man she had ever made love to had been her husband and for the most part she had gotten nothing out of it except the holding and the talking.

Mary eased Weld's head off her lap so she could get a blanket to cover him with. The fire had died down and it was getting chilly.

How terrible for Weld to have lost both parents in one day. She remembered her own grief and again shed tears of loss. She called Vera to stoke the fire and to put in more wood. Weld slept through the entire day waking only long enough to visit the bathroom, take a drink of water and hold Mary's hand for a moment. When he awoke at five p.m. he was flustered for a moment, not knowing where he was.

"I'm so sorry Mary. I didn't intend to fall asleep."

"It's all right," she told him. "I know how it feels to lose your loved ones. I've been there."

"I must go. The family will be worried. I've been gone nine hours and I had intended to go right back to the farm," Weld worried.

He stood by the door his hat in his hand wishing he could hold her for a moment, but he had only known her for a twenty four hour period and most of that he had slept.

When he drove into the yard Henry came to meet him. "We were about ta go look fer ya," he said. "Did ya run into some kind of problem?"

"No, I just went ta say hello ta a friend and I fell asleep." Weld explained.

"A lady friend, at this time?" Henry sarcastically inquired.

"No, not that kind a thing. I just felt I could not move another inch without a little time out. I had not understood how out of it I was and I just went ta sleep."

"We had better go inside so everyone can see ya are all in one piece," Henry urged.

Weld had to relate to everyone what had happened again.

The lawyer, Mr. Wiley was at the farm with the legal papers and the will which he wanted to get started reading now that all were present.

The will read in essence, "We, Abby and Jacob Winter, being of sound mind, etc. etc. Further on into the will the family was instructed to wait one year before making plans about what to do about the farm permanently when everyone would be less emotionally disturbed. The money on hand was to be divided equally between the sons and Raye. The young children have money in trust to raise them on and for them to have control of when they reached the ages of twenty one. Our hopes are that one or all of you will take care of Harriet, Mildred and Rosie until they marry or become of age.

There is a separate account for the farm expenditures at the bank. Continue to deposit surplus income into that account each month. Use it as it is needed to run the farm. If after one year, none of the family wants to keep the farm sell it and all the livestock, pay off any debts then divide the money equally between all surviving family members.

If any family member or members wish to take over the farm for themselves, take out a loan on the farm and pay off the remaining family members. You will find a list amongst the papers that designate pieces of furniture, knickknacks and such that go to different family members. Leave them in the house until or if you sell. All monies are deposited at the bank. Mr. Wiley has a record of how much just as the bank has. There was a codicil to the will added after they had received the artwork from Lizzet. The portrait can rest in a different family member's homes each year. The statuette is Weld's to do with as he decides.

All of our family, children, in-laws and other relations are dear to us. Try to give each other the benefit of the doubt. If tempers flare, back off and think things over. Never fight or argue. We know each of you and every one of you is a person to be proud of.

Signed, Abby Winter and Jacob Winter and dated.

Everyone sat silent thinking how wise and giving their parents had been. They were all so glad not to have to make decisions. Now each felt as if the weight of the world had been lifted from them.

Supper tonight consisted of leftovers with plenty of cold milk and coffee.

Weld took over the cooking for the family and the hands. He had been right when he had told his mother that he was a good cook. Everybody always slicked their plates clean no matter what he served.

Raye kept the little girls on weekends, and Jerry and Carly took them from time to time. They all helped with laundry, sometimes taking the clothes to their houses, sometimes coming to the farm to do it.

The girls divided the house cleaning. One came on Monday, a different one on Wednesday and another on Friday. Weld kept the kitchen ship shape, dishes and all. He put in several hours a day doing farm labor along with the rest of the hands. He had been pushed into taking over Jacob's duties. He was lining out the work, making payroll and doing the shopping. He also got the younguns off to school. He got their dinner pails packed teeth checked, clean dresses and shoelaces tied.

Tonight Weld had informed everyone, "I'm gone fer the night and maybe longer. Don't look fer me 'til ya see me comin'." As he took off he whistled happily.

Mary was very glad to see him. She had been very concerned about him since she had last seen him. Her heart skipped a beat when he smiled.

"Howdy!" he said. "Can ya take pity on a poor ol' lonesome cowboy and have supper with him?" he begged.

"I think that could be arranged, unless that cowboy would like to take supper here. I don't cook but Vera is a fantastic cook." She smiled.

"Done!" Weld said, kissing her lightly on the cheek. He wanted to grab her up and swing her around but he contained him self. Her lips were full and looked soft and luscious. Yes, he really wanted to hold her and kiss her, but he knew instinctively she was a good and moral woman and he must not take advantage of her sweetness.

The food was great, cooked and seasoned just right. Yes Vera was a good cook.

After they had finished eating she invited him into the parlor, where he had slept all day that second day after so much sadness. He could remember her smoothing his hair and touching his face talking softly to him telling him things would get better in time. Maybe he should let her take the lead and see where things might go.

They sat side by side, talking for hours she told him of her horror of the never ending pain and how she missed her child and her husband's arms. Slowly she inched closer to Weld asking if he would like to kiss her.

"At this moment I don't believe I've ever wanted anything so badly as I want ta hold ya and kiss ya."

She lifted her lips to his. Weld jerked, it felt as if an electric shock had struck him. Evidently it was the same for her because she drew back to look into his eyes. She then put both arms around his neck and clung to him, holding his lips with hers, never wanting to let go. They were both shaking and breathless still needing to be closer and closer.

Weld attempted to draw back and loose her arms from his neck, but she held even tighter. “Mary, we can’t do this. I’ll be going back ta California shortly and I don’t want to mislead ya in any way.”

She just held tighter, imprisoning his lips with hers. He became lost in her sweetness and forgot everything else wanting more and more of her. Before he realized what was happening she had all but one of his shirt buttons undone.

“No, no. Please, ya must stop. I can’t take any more just now.” Finally he grabbed both her wrists, holding her away from him. “Mary, we cannot, we must not. I’m not ready ta get married. I have many responsibilities.

“I understand,” she admitted. “But now is now and I want you with all of me. No strings attached.”

Still he tried to back away but his body had taken over his mind. He had to have her, every bit of her. He swept her up into his arms and lay her gently on the bed. For a moment Dottie flashed through his mind. They had no agreement or even an understanding. They were both free agents but he really did like Dottie. But at that moment with Mary here, wanting and willing he just could not stop. He could tell Mary had never been made love to as he was making love to her now. She was holding his head to her lips and later to her breast. She arched and moved herself against him. She was now experiencing emotions she had not known existed. It was wonderful. They lay marveling at the glorious feelings even now that lingered.

Weld held her, kissed her and spoke sweet love words to her and she began to kiss him back. She was like a starved puppy trying to taste everything at once. “Wait, wait.” Weld told her. “Give us a little time. Let’s wash up have something to drink, juice, coffee or milk,” he said.

She told Weld, “I’ve been married three years of my life, but I have never had these feelings before.”

Later the performance was repeated but at a more leisurely pace. Weld made love to her for hours. She was such a sweet and loving person he wanted to make the experience a lovely one for her. Later both completely exhausted they feel asleep entwined in each other’s arms.

Weld awoke to the smell of bacon and coffee. Mary had been up for two hours. She had let him sleep but thought, “After he eats and builds up some strength he will be mine again if I can manage it." She was so happy and content for the first time since her baby and his father had been killed.

Weld ate every scrap of food in sight. He was ravenous. The food was good and the company superb. He felt great. There was nothing like a woman to put life back into him. Women were God's greatest creation.

They sat in the parlor and she had coffee. No matter how good coffee smelled Weld preferred milk and lots of it.

Mary sat next to Weld, cuddled up close to him tracing his lips with her fingers, nipping at his ears and neck. He opened the buttons of her blouse all the way down and unhooked her skirt. Picking her up they went into the bedroom locking the door behind them. He didn't know where Vera was or what her schedule was to clean the rooms but he did not want an audience. Every fiber of his being was throbbing with passion.

"Hold me! Please just hold me." He did.

"Weld, I'm in love with you." Mary said. "I know you are not the marrying kind. I agree to what you said, no strings, no regrets, only love me while you are here. I'll hold it for the rest of my life."

Weld held her close, kissing her telling her how wonderful she was and how wonderful she made him feel. He told her of how he loved being with her making love to her, smelling her scent and feeling her soft flesh pressed against him. "Ya make me happy through and through," he swore.

Weld had been gone from the ranch twenty six hours. He guessed he needed to go home but he really didn't want to go.

"Not yet! Please not yet." Mary begged. "Love me again!" she pleaded. "Once more. Please!"

Mary wanted to get a strong chain and lock Weld to the metal bedpost so he could never leave but she knew she had to let him go or he would run and never return. Maybe he would miss her enough to stay or to take her with him even if he wouldn't marry her. She would take whatever he could give her.

Weld dragged into the farm at nine p.m. Just in time for bed.

Henry and Jack hoo-rahed him telling him he looked just like a mouse the cat had drug in. Weld just shook his head slightly and smiled.

Next morning Weld made breakfast for everyone. There were a little less tension and sorrows, even a few smiles shown forth.

Weld had sent Bob full details on how everything had happened and the copies of the will and the other legal papers, money, everything. He didn't know just how long it was going to take for everyone to get in step, so to speak, but not too soon as it looked now. "Ya might want ta think about if ya would ever want ta come back here or work on the farm. We have all discussed it, none deciding anything. Ya know wives, their families, too much pressure, want ta see the world, too young. I've heard it all. I'll be needin' yer vote by a year from now, think on it.

Weld wasn't sure he wanted to spend his life on the Bar-X-Z. He liked the work and the people but ranching kept a man very busy. You didn't have time for much of anything else. His feet just sometimes get itchy and he needs to go someplace nowhere in particular just someplace new. There are too many people needing too much of your time he thought. Oh he would never take off if his family really needed him but he was going to have to show Henry and Jack how to fend for themselves. They had to learn to cook and sew and do laundry too. The sisters in law and Raye already have plenty to do at their own homes. When he went home, Weld reasoned there would be no one to do it for them.

At supper Weld brought up the subject to Jack and Henry. "Cook? Me cook?" They both shouted, "I ain't cookin'!"

"Well, ya can always starve or hire a cook. That'll cost ya more than ya make working all day," Weld offered.

Jack and Henry grumbled and said "No way!"

That night Jack and Henry asked Weld, "How long ya got before ya have ta leave?"

"I've got one more month before I have ta leave. I have everything lined out here. The lawyer Mr. Wiley, has all the papers and records of everything. The only thing missing is a way ta feed ya and the extra hands. Did ya ever ask if one of the new hands can cook? If so then work them half day and let them take care of cooking and kitchen cleaning the other half. Give them two hours fer breakfast and dishes, let them work fer four hours then two hours fer supper and dishes. One of ya will have ta keep the beds made and changed and the house picked up. Ya will need ta carry in wood and water, milk and gather eggs and the washing and ironing of your clothes."

"Damn!" The boys said. "We can't do that woman stuff."

"Sure ya can or ya can do without."

Weld knew they would never be able to keep their jobs and keep the house up. He called a meeting with everyone present and put forth the problem. "Shall we hire a housekeeper cook charged to the farm or can ya figure a way to feed the hands keep the younguns taken care of and that sorta thing?"

"We just thought ya would take care of it 'til the year was up," Jerry said.

"Boys, I own a third interest in a thousand acre ranch. Bob is just helpin' me out. I have a home, just like the rest of ya. Besides in a year it will still be the same so we must decide now. Go home, talk it over and let me know."

Weld put out notice they were looking for an all around housekeeper, cook. They hoped to find a lady of forty or perhaps a little older. Someone strong and easy going that could fix good plain food and live in. We will pay five dollars over the going wage per month.

Three different ladies applied for the job the second day but they just weren't quite right. On the fourth day a lady named Grace asked to see the person looking to hire a housekeeper, cook. She was shown into the kitchen where Weld was preparing two large hens for baking. He rose as she entered the room saying, "howdy Ma'am, may I be of help ta ya?"

"Probably, but right now I think I might be of more help to you," she stated. "My name is Grace White. I'm here about the housekeeper, cook job. Here let me do that while we talk." She took the hen right out of his hands saying, "I need a job. I have no place to stay. My husband died and my father in law tossed me out. I'm a fine cook and I keep a clean house. I like younguns and I ain't lazy. I don't drink or curse and I don't chase around. I've never worked for anyone except myself my husband and his mean ol' Dad. What else do you want to know?"

"Oh, I think that's a plenty Grace. When can ya start?"

"I just did," she said. "Now if you'll show me where everything is, I'll get things started. What time is supper? How many at each meal? How old are the younguns and do they eat at the same time as the rest of the family? Breakfast is at six a.m. I take it."

"Breakfast is at six thirty a.m. supper at six p.m. The younguns eat supper with the family and breakfast at seven thirty. The girls are eleven, nine and four, I think, but ya better check that out with them. Mama mostly home schooled them and all the rest of us, but they have been going ta school fer a while now."

"Well I ain't the best English teacher but I do well on sums. Mostly I spell like I talk, but I could hone up on spelling if need be."

"I believe our sister, Raye, wants ta be a teacher and intends teachin' them in the coldest months," Weld allowed.

"Where do I sleep?" Grace asked.

"Top of the stairs second door on the left," Weld informed her.

"What do I call all of you? Mr. Winter or by your given name?"

“My name is Weld, the youngest brother is Henry and the other one is Jack. Ya can ask the hired hands what they will answer to. The vegetable house fer the canned foods is out the door and ta the left. The cellar is ta its left and the smoke house is ta the right next ta the well. The chicken houses are toward the barn on the south. Besides the chicken houses, the hens lay in the barn. Fresh eggs are stored on the right and the older eggs are kept on the left in the cellar. We don’t want the fresh eggs ta be eaten or sold before the ones that go ta market every Saturday. Just nose around ta find the things ya need. Ever three ta four months we gather up the non-laying hens and can up as many as ya think we will need and every eight weeks we sell off the fryers we don’t need ta eat. Hens are settin’ all the time except December and January, they don’t set much in the cold weather. I think we have around two thousand chickens most of the time. The hands take care of the chickens and all the animals, including egg gathering and storage. Mama always warned us not ta leave the canned vegetables door opened. She said light was what caused most folks canned stuff ta spoil,” Weld informed Grace.

“She was right!” Grace agreed.

When the hands came to supper everything smelled wonderful. There was chicken and dressing and chicken and dumplings. They smelled fresh bread and pie. Everyone, including Weld agreed that Grace was a superb cook.

Weld told Grace, "You're a better cook than I am. Welcome and I hope we all get along together.

At five forty five a.m. Weld heard Grace leave her room. Minutes later he smelled coffee and bacon. When he went down to the kitchen, Grace was putting biscuits into the oven. A kettle on the middle stove lids was bubbling along full of oatmeal. The huge frying pan was full of bacon and eggs set ready to fry. "How many eggs do I need to cook? I don't know how many eggs each of you usually eat."

The Winter boys each ate three eggs, three biscuits, six bacon strips, a large bowl of oats, milk, juice and coffee. The hired hands, which were heavier than any of the Winters', ate much less but stayed heavy. Abby and Jacob had been big eaters but had never gained an ounce.

Friday evening, Weld took off again. I won't be back until Sunday noon, or around then," he told the family and Grace.

Mary was doing her act when Weld walked in. he caught her eye and nodded toward the back. She dipped her chin down and Weld went back out the door and around to the side door where he knocked and was admitted by Vera.

Weld had brought fresh food from the farm. He had beef, chicken, eggs, fresh milk, canned fruit and nuts. Vera took them and he could hear her getting out pans and he soon smelled the wonderful aroma of mixed foods cooking.

Mary came into her apartment running to Weld, kissing him all over his face.

"Whoa, slow down baby. I'm yours until Sunday," Weld promised. "I brought food from the farm. Vera is preparing supper for us."

"I still have a show to do later tonight," Mary wailed.

"That's fine. I'll either leave a few minutes before you do and take a seat at the bar so I can watch ya on stage or I can rest up here if that's all right with ya." Weld promised.

"Anything you do is fine with me as long as you spend all your time with me," she said pulling at his shirtfront.

"Easy now, remember Vera, supper, daylight is far off. We have a lot of time. I've thought about ya almost every minute" he assured her. "I can't get ya out of my mind."

"Me too," she said. "I dream of you making love to me."

****

CHAPTER 22

Bob spent much of his waking hours on horseback, just riding and talking to Socks, remembering his yesteryears with the family. Now Mama and Papa were gone. He wished he had stayed at home, never leaving the farm. Maybe things would have been different and maybe Papa would not have been handling that stallion and Mama would still be there. "Damn! Damn!" he said aloud.

He had thought he might stay on in California and maybe take up law so he could help those who have so little. Bureaucrats just seemed so heartless or maybe they just did not realize how hopeless a person feels with no work, no food and no place to live. When a parent looks at a child crying for something to eat, when they are unable to fill this child's stomach, it has to eat at them constantly. Now he just couldn't get his mind straight on what to do or where to do it.

Another thing, there was Julie. She had become very important to him. He admired her enjoyed being with her and wanted her so badly he could not think straight when he was near her or even just thinking of her as he was now. Damn!

Gladys had offered to let him take off and go home saying she, Jake and Slade and the rest of the hands could take care of the ranch for a couple of months. He had considered it but then had declined. He had made a deal with Weld. He would stay until Weld returned come what may.

Suddenly he was aware of cattle moving fast down from the north of where he now sat astride Socks. He cocked his head to the right trying to locate just where the sound was coming from. He then saw about a hundred head being driven hard by four men cracking whips behind the herd. Bob got down from Socks' back, withdrawing his rifle and loosening his holstered gun. He dropped behind a huge boulder took careful aim at the rider closest to him and fired. The man fell off his horse crying, "I've been shot, help me!" one fellow came to his aid but the other two kept with the herd. Again Bob drew careful aim and knocked one of the men from their horse. The fourth man slowed and looked trying to locate Bob his gun in his hand. Bob raised his rifle aimed for the rider's gun hand and fired. He saw the gun fly from the man's hand. The hand was hanging loosely at the man's side dripping blood.

Bob stepped into view asking the four men to drop their gun belts and move in together where he could see them all more easily. “I am a Marshall and I’m placin’ ya all under arrest fer cattle russlin.” He told them. He cut four short lengths of rope from his lariat telling one of them to tie the other three tightly then he tied the fourth man.

“Ya know fellers, I coulda killed all of ya so ya best give some thought ta changin’ yer ways. If this were a few years ago ya would just be strung up without a trial. However we now have laws that handle this sort of thing. He tied a rope through their horse’s bridles then looped the ropes tightly around each of their waists, taking them tied together with the rope looped over his saddle horn. “Now fellers, keep at a walk or ya will be walkin’ on foot and I will shoot ya if I have ta.”

Riding into the yard the hands gathered around. Bob gave them the details and sent Slade into town for the sheriff. The men were locked in the granary. There were no windows in the sturdy building. The door was locked and Jake sat rifle in hand, guarding the door.

Bob went inside and reported to Gladys. “My goodness! Who are they?” Gladys asked.

"Never seen um before." Bob said, "But we need ta send some men ta check the fences. They must have a hole cut someplace ta run the cattle through."

Slade and the sheriff drove up in separate automobiles. Bob came out giving the sheriff the information and leading him to the granary, where Jake still sat his rifle across his knees.

When the door was opened the sheriff smiled saying, "We are old acquaintances. These are the four Samson brothers. I've been lookin' fer 'em. They stole a herd of horses from a feller 'bout ten miles to the south. They wuz recognized but we just miss 'em ever place we go. Come on boys. We go a date with the hoosegow in town." The sheriff said leading them towards the hands that were to accompany the sheriff into town on horseback.

Bob was a natural when it came to applying the law. Always before, he had never had to fire his gun at anyone. Now he had wounded three men and one horse. The horse only slightly where the bullet went through the first man's leg and scratched the horse, but the animal was fine.

Bob sat down and wrote Weld a long letter telling how everything on Bar-X-Z was progressing including the episode with the rustlers. "I'm getting restless Weld. How soon will you be back?" he asked. "I'm not sure what I'm going to do but I need the freedom to make that choice which I cannot do under these circumstances. My heart breaks every time I think of Mama and Papa which is almost constantly. I don't know if I'm going to be able to have closure until I actually go back home and see everything for myself. I know you and the boys are taking care of everything but I just can't stop thinking I need to do something myself. I know it would not have changed anything if I had been there but I feel so guilty. Except for Julie I would have no problem going back to stay on the farm, but there is Julie. I'll figure it all out," he said, closing with Love Bob.

Julie was aware of Bob's affection for her. She liked and respected Bob more than anyone else she knew, but she was not in love with him nor could she ever be. It was his brother Weld she yearned for who had never given her a glance. The very first time she saw Weld Winter she knew if she ever married it would be Weld, or no one.

Gladys had figured it out Julie thought, knowing how often she asked about Weld, not Bob. Julie tried very hard not to encourage Bob but they worked together so much serving the homeless it was hard not to lean on him in emergencies. He was so involved in the movement and his heart was as big as the whole world and he had a need to give of himself in every way possible. She was going to let him think she was involved with one of the guys in her social circle starting today. Once having made up her mind she didn't hesitate when Bob ask her to have dinner with him.

"Oh Bob, I'm sorry! I've made plans to be with my boy friend Fred. He hates me spending so much time here but he is a dear about it." She smiled. "Some other time maybe," she offered.

Bob felt his whole body sag. He just wilted like an orchid in the sun. He had just assumed she felt as he did. "I guess I'll go on then and get a bite," he said. Turning, he stumbled toward Ma's Place but his appetite was gone. "Well, that takes care of that," he thought. "Now I can return to Kansas just as soon as Weld gets here."

Bob went to the telegraph office and sent a telegram to Weld. “Coming home -stop- Gladys and hands will care for ranch—stop- things for me changed.—stop- Bob.

Bob talked to Gladys explaining that he just had to go and that he would not be back but that Weld would be home very soon.

Gladys felt she knew what had happened but said nothing. She had no worries about the ranch. The way Weld had everything set up it could almost run itself. They had good hands, honest and each know what to do without any coaching. Of course she would be glad to have Weld back. He was like a son to her.

Julie went home alone and cried. She really did care for Bob she just did not love him. She hoped he went back to his people. There are people in every city that need help.

He would find his niche amongst his neighborhood needy and shortly he would find someone he could enjoy being with again.

Weld showed the telegram to Mary whose face turned ashen. “Now don’t go getting’ all upset.” Weld comforted her. “I’ll introduce ya ta Bob when he gets here. He is gonna need a lot of comforting and you are the one ta help him. Just never mention anything about knowin' me in any way except socially. He will love ya just as I do and give ya the love ya need as well," he assured her.

"But Weld, I love you, not your brother. I can't just turn my love off and turn it on for another."

"Wrong! Ya don't love me. Ya want me just as I do ya. We make crazy love like ya have never known before. Now ya can enjoy making love with almost anyone. Just choose men that don't talk. Never meet in the saloon. Keep it private. Weld instructed, "And never admit ta any man, that there has ever been anyone else. They will protect your name. Now how about some sweet lovin' right now?" he wheedled.

Before he even got the words out she was at him like a mountain lion. She was tearing at his buttons and running her hands all over him catching his tongue between her teeth. She kissed him furiously as if there would never be another kiss, or arms to hold her again.

Weld thought, "Since this woman had been awakened she is fire." Never had he made love to a woman who had satisfied him as she did. Mary took great delight in arousing Weld. She could do it so easily and so well.

"Come here! Come here!" he groaned. "I love ta kiss ya baby. Love me while I love ya."

"How was he going to leave her for Bob or anyone else?" he wondered. "She is like wine in my soul. I could never stay around here and not have her."

He would be leaving tomorrow after Bob arrived. He intended to introduce him to Mary at the little eating place next to the saloon. Mary would be seated alone looking very demure he would insist on a snack before they went to the farm. He would leave the rest to Mary and Mother Nature.

As they walked through the door, Bob noticed Mary right away. "What a beautiful woman!" he said.

"Would ya like ta meet her?" Weld asked.

"Sure would!" Bob replied.

Weld stopped at Mary's table taking his hat off, asking if he might introduce his brother.

"I would be delighted." Mary said, smiling that wonderful smile.

"Bob, may I present Miss Mary. She owns Mary's next door. Mary, this is my brother Bob," Weld said.

Mary saw the same tenderness in Bob's eyes as in Weld's. When he bent to kiss her hand shocks like lightning ran through her. Bob too felt the shock. "May I call on ya sometime after I get settled?" he inquired.

"Would you please?" she answered. When she arose to leave she winked at Weld.

Everyone was waiting to see Bob. They were throwing their arms around him, patting him on the back, crying and talking about their parents, how they missed them and if only, etc. etc.

Bob had been gone from home for almost four years. He had matured and grown into a man since he had left.

Weld had told Bob before he caught the train out at the depot that he would go along with whatever the family decided but that Bob might think on running the farm or buying out one or more of the boys if he decided to stay on.

The three young girls had grown so much he would never have known them if they had been mixed up in a group. They had about forgotten him as well but in a few days it was, do you remember this? Or, how about the time that…and so on. They felt just like old times.

Bob loved his mother's portrait. He stood looking at it for a long time. "The artist had really seen the inner Abby as well as thee outer one," he marveled. The sculpture of Weld was also very good indeed. It was so lifelike you nearly expected it to speak.

The stallion that had killed Jacob had been sold with a warning to be very careful around him. He was a good stallion but they couldn't stand to see him around the barn. They had replaced him with one just as good and a lot less dangerous.

Bob was introduced to Grace the cook telling her his food intake would be the same as Weld's. They were all hungry men who enjoyed food in abundance.

"You look like Weld. Do you cook as well?"

"Oh I've been known ta rattle a skillet at times. Why?"

"Are you better than Weld?" she asked.

"Nope! Weld is the cook of the family," Bob admitted. "Why?"

"Just needed to know if I had any competition" she laughed. "Weld said I could out cook him, so I guess I'm safe," she laughed.

She served up a roast piglet with cinnamon apples glazed over with maple syrup, sweet potatoes, a huge green salad, green squash and sautéed mushrooms, biscuits, fresh churned butter and chocolate layer cake. Everything was delicious and beautiful to look at.

"Grace, ya are the best. Ya have no competition," Bob agreed.

Everyone just expected Bob to take over make the decisions and make the farm produce at a net gain. Bob looked everything over. He couldn't see anything that needed changed. Weld had everything laid out and operating at a good percent.

Weld had left all the legal papers, ledgers, banking etc. for Bob, all in order. No monies had been dispersed to any of the Winter family. They had all voted not to divide the cash on hand for the year when everything was to be divided or try to decide what had to be done about it.

Bob was given the itinerary as to when eggs, fryers and hens were to be taken to market. He said to continue just as they had been.

His horse was back in California so he chose a shiny black mare with a white mane and tail. She was full of pep, but handled nicely.

He dropped the reins and guided her with his knees when he dropped the reins to the ground she stopped and didn't attempt to leave. "She would do," he thought, taking off at a good fast gallop. She was a smooth animal. He named her Jet.

Henry and Jack rode up beside him grinning. "How are ya feelin' brother Bob?" Jackson asked him.

"I'm still tired from the trip and the emotional lick still has me reelin', but I'll be fine," he said.

"Have ya been thinkin' on what we should be plannin' fer next year? Ya know, do ya think ya want ta stay on the farm, or sell out?"

Jack said. "I been thinkin' along those lines before the accident," he admitted. "I think maybe I'd like ta check out the railroad or maybe leave out on a good ship. I don't suppose I'll stay with it but I want the experience. Ya know how I've always read everything I can git my hands on about trains and ships. How about ya Henry?"

"I don't know. I guess I don't have a goal yet. I know I always want ta work outside in the fresh air and sunshine. I'm not ready ta settle down, don't want a wife or kids yet and maybe never. I guess I'll just coast fer a while," Henry stated.

Weld asked, "Do either of ya want ta sell yer share of the farm or do ya want ta keep it and go try out the fantasies?"

Jack said, "I'll probably sell or give my share ta whoever takes over. I know fer sure I don't want ta be a farmer."

"I'm just staying fer a while," Henry said. "I'll figure it out by the time allotted."

"Have ya heard anything from the married boys or Raye?"

"Raye wants ta be a teacher but she also made mention of takin' the younguns ta raise. However I don't know what Haskins will say about that. He is a good man and a good farmer. He knows his stuff so ta speak."

"Jerry's wife, don't like fer him ta spend so much time workin'. She needs a lot of attention and she likes ta go ta the social gatherings. I think he will vote ta sell."

Frank has already bought another three hundred acres and is runnin' cattle along with grain and hay crops to feed through the winter. I heard him wishin' the year was up or that he could git some of the cash Mama and Papa had left each of us so he could pay off his land. So I'd say he wants ta sell too." Henry replied.

“Carl just wants enough money ta get his dairy on pay ground he always said he was gonna have the best dairy around when he grew up. It’s his dream.”

“Well I guess that’s about half and half.” Bob said. “Cept fer me and Weld. Really just me. Weld says he doesn’t care which way we vote but he won’t be comin’ back here ta live. He has too much tied up in the Bar-X-Z. Not just money. It allows him freedom ta travel which is his first love. I like seein’ new places and meetin’ new people as well. Being Marshall affords me that pleasure. But I want a home base fer when I’m not on the go, lookin’ fer someone. I think I’d like ta buy out some of ya. Maybe Raye, Patrick and the younguns and I could get along on the farm, livin’ under the same roof. The three girls were left trust funds for when they are grown but are ta be taken care of until then from proceeds from the farm.

“I reckon I’ll speak ta the boys find out their thoughts right now. If anyone needs money right now, I think that can be arranged. If anyone wants ta sell their share now, I think I can come up with the money. I’m definitely staying with the farm,” Bob declared.

Bob got the automobile and drove by and picked up Carl and Frank then stopped at Jerry's.

"Howdy boys. What do ya need?" Jerry asked.

"Just a pow wow." Bob told him. "I've come ta inquire if any or all of you would like ta receive your money from the folks now and ta find out if ya intend ta stay doin' what ya are doin' now, or do ya think ya would like ta run the farm? Ya know be responsible for the running of it and the paying to each holder, do the books. Ya know the whole ball of wax."

Jerry spoke first. "I definitely do not want ta run the farm. I want ta farm my own land and do what I'm doin' now. I vote ta sell."

Carl looked around him. "I need money now. I also vote ta sell."

"I'd like ta be able ta pay off my land," Frank said. "I vote ta sell as well.

"I've talked ta Henry and Jackson. Henry hasn't made up his mind yet and Jackson doesn't care one way or the other. But he wants ta leave the farm ta look into railroads and ships. He is ready ta go now. I'll speak ta Raye and Patick then I'll get back ta ya." Bob promised.

"Has anyone thought ta have the farm appraised?" Bob wanted to know.

"Don't think so." Jerry offered.

"Well, we will get that done and I'll see if I can get enough money together ta buy ya out. I'm staying!" Bob stated. "I also must send Jenny a cablegram fer her vote." He said.

Raye was making bread, flour on her hands and her cute little nose. Bob broached the subject of her and Patrick moving into the farmhouse and renting out their farm, taking care of the girls and living there together with him.

She said, "I know I will need to care for the girls. I also know this house is not nearly large enough and we hope to have children of our own but it will be entirely up to Patrick. I would never force him into any situation especially when or how he makes our living. That is his domain entirely. As for my self, yes it sounds like the only practical solution. The girls need a steady, safe life.

He told Raye of the boy's thoughts on the situation and his intention of purchasing their shares.

Bob went into town to send word to Jenny. He sent, "All want to sell except me and Henry—stop- want your vote—stop- Raye takes children—stop- I buy out boys—stop- Your share?—stop- Bob."

He sent an identical one to Weld.

Now he stood at the bar at Mary's Place listening to her beautiful voice, watching that gorgeous body sway to the music. "How beautiful she is," he thought. Bob sent a note to her, asking to see her. She sent Vera out with an invitation and instructions to go to the side door in twenty minutes.

He wondered what kind of entertainment she liked and what kind of foods she would enjoy. When Vera opened the door, he stood there with a single red rose in his hand.

"Oh madam loves roses," she informed Bob. "Come this way," she invited. He could smell something delicious from the kitchen. It smelled like apple pie and roast pork, if his nose wasn't lying to him.

Mary came through the door from the back of the room. She looked radiant, happy, glowing. "Hello Mr. Winter," she smiled. "I hope you will dine with me. I have a second show in two hours."

"Thank you," he said handing her the rose.

"Oh how beautiful!" she said, holding it to her nose. "Roses are my favorite flowers. Come." She patted the seat beside her. "Sit here so I can see your eyes when we speak. I'm a fanatic about looking into the eyes of the person I'm speaking to. Where have you been for the last few years? Weld said you had just gotten in after a few years."

"I've been ta quite a few places, most recently California. I'm going ta be staying now on the Winter Farm," he told her.

Vera had placed on a small round table with a white cloth over it, very tempting fare. It consisted of, steaming roast pork, baked potatoes, green peas, sliced tomatoes, salad and apple pie.

Bob held the chair for Mary. She leaned her head to the left just enough to brush her cheek against his fingers sending a thrill through him and herself as well.

They ate talked and laughed through the meal. She took his hand as they left the table leading him to the settee, pulling him close to her side of the seat. She looked into his eyes invitingly but he didn't take the bait. He knew women's eyes often said one thing then changed to another.

"It's almost time for my next performance," she pouted. "Would you care to wait here until I've finished or do you have other things to do?"

"I have nothing important to do but are ya sure ya want me ta stay?"

"Very sure."

Bob took off his boots and stretched out on the settee. He didn't know how long she might be gone so he took off his jacket as well. Bob had fallen asleep almost as soon as his head hit the pillow that rested on the end of the seat. He dreamed of Julie of making love to her when he had never so much as kissed her.

Mary came in seeing Bob resting, his boots and jacket lay on a chair. She carefully disrobed putting on nothing except a clinging robe that exposed most of her breast and gaped open when she moved. "If this doesn't clue him in he is dense," she thought.

She told Vera to retire for the night that she would not be needed before morning. Hearing her voice, Bob awoke. He reached for his boots but Mary let the robe fall to the floor, reaching for Bob's buttons.

"My how flawless her skin is and that body is enough ta run a man crazy," Bob thought. Bob didn't have the knack that Weld had to be relaxed and make the first move until he knew for sure just what the game was. When he knew though he took charge pretty much as Weld had. He was somewhat larger than Weld, all over.

Like Weld, he continued to hold her whispering sweet nothings into her ear, kissing her softly and telling her how wonderful she was.

It was almost daylight when Bob dressed and went home. She had asked him if he would come back again. He smiled, "Just try to keep me away."

Just like with Weld, they hoo-rahed Bob for being out all night and dragging in just before breakfast. He didn't mind at all. He had, had the best night of his life and plenty more to come. He sang and whistled all day as he worked.

Bob received word from both Jenny and Weld, each saying about the same thing. "You keep my part—stop- money and farm—stop- take care of children—stop- letter follows—stop-"

That meant only Jerry, Frank and Carl would be selling their shares. Henry hadn't decided yet. The money each of them would receive from the sale of the farm in total would amount to approximately twelve thousand five hundred dollars, or the total Bob had to come up with of forty five thousand dollars. With Weld and Jenny's part of the value of the farm and their part of the cash he could almost pay the boys off right now. That included of course his money from the gold coins and what he had added to it from his salary. The lawyer had gotten everything counted. The cash to each was ten thousand dollars, plus one ninth the value of the farm came to seventeen thousand dollars each. With his ten thousand, Weld's ten and Jenny's ten, he could pay thirty thousand plus his savings. He would have to give them a contract to pay off each of their shares of the balance owed if they would agree.

Bob told about Weld and Jenny turning their shares over to him if he would stay on the farm, keeping a home for the little girls until they were grown. I can pay each of you thirteen thousand now and give you a note to pay off the balance paid monthly or bi-monthly.

Jerry spoke up and offered to accept the thirteen thousand as payment in full as his contribution for the care of the children. Frank and Carl echoed Jerry's statement.

“I’ll get the money tomorrow,” Bob said.

Bob now owned six of the nine shares of the farm or two thirds, without having to make payments. He knew his commitment was for at least twelve years or more, until the children were grown. “I can do it,” he said to himself, “with a little time off once in awhile to take on a special case for the state.” He went around singing, thinking of Mary.

A letter came from Weld with notarized statements giving Bob his share of the farm and his share of the money. Everything was falling right into place.

The farm was in good shape with the cattle in good health and increasing. The chickens and the other animals couldn’t be expected to do any better than they were.

Patrick and Raye came to the farm Friday for supper. They informed everyone at the table they had talked it over and decided they would indeed move onto the farm and care for the children. They would also run cattle on their own farm, renting out only the house and five acres. They already had a renter.

Patrick told Bob, “I won’t have anything to do with the running of the farm. I’ll just work as a hand drawing a salary same as the others.”

“If that’s the way ya want it,” Bob agreed.

Jackson said I guess I’ll be taking off next week. Just deposit my share of the cash into my account at the bank. I won’t be needing money from the farm, just use that ta help care for the girls.”

Henry piped up. “The same for me. I’ve decided ta keep Jack company. I might like trains or ships. At least for a while.”

“Ya know, I coulda used a little more notice ta find more hands,” Bob said.

“Oh we will give ya time fer that. We may even know some fellers that want ta work.

“I just don’t think they can stand to be apart,” Raye said. “They have always been so close.”

A letter was waiting for Bob when he got in from riding fence. It was from Jenny. She had sent the same signed papers as Weld had done. “I have all the money I will ever need and I surely will not ever be moving back to Kansas and we want to help with the small ones.”

She wrote. She went on to tell him how big James Jacob was getting and how his father doted on him. “He will be the most spoiled boy in the world. Oh and that thing with Gilly and Paul has played out. I guess he finally wised up. For awhile I thought she had her claws into him so far he would never get away.”

“My business is doing well. Much better than I could ever have imagined. My designs are in shops all over Europe and America now. I’m really lucky. James keeps very busy at Arltons. Peg has turned over most of the business end to him. He likes keeping busy. Write me a long letter giving me all the news.” Love Jenny.

****

CHAPTER 23

Weld stopped at Dottie's before he went on to the ranch. She wasn't as happy to see him as he had thought she would be. In fact, she was not happy at all. He was stupefied.

"I've met someone, who unlike you wants to marry me." She told him. We have not had sex but I can teach him if he does not know how to make love."

"I'm happy for you Dottie but I advise ya ta try before ya buy. Some people, men or women won't participate in what many see as sinful," Weld warned her. He kissed her cheek and left. Weld was surprised to hear Dottie wanted to be married. She had said she would never marry again. "Everyone changes their mind sometime," He thought.

When he started for a driver rig he ran into Julie. She was beautifully dressed as usual. Her eyes shone with happiness when she saw Weld. "I didn't know you were back. When did you get home?"

"I've not been home yet. I just got in," he explained. "Would ya care ta have a snack or somethin' while I'm waiting for a driver ta take me out ta the ranch."

"If you would allow me I'd love ta drive ya home," Julie offered.

"Great, I'd like that and we could talk. How is the project ta help the needy comin' along? Have the town Father's fallen into line at all?"

"No it's all strictly volunteer but we are better organized now. We have portioned off areas with certain groups to take care of specific areas Gladys and I still have the lion's share at our neighborhood. Gladys is such a dear, always ready to do anything she can. The milk, eggs and chicken from the Bar-X-Z is a God send."

Julie pulled into the drive at the front of the house just as Jake and Slade stepped off the porch. Spotting Weld beside Julie they reached for his hand welcoming him home.

"It's been quite a while Weld said and so much has happened but I'm glad ta be back. How are things goin' here?" he asked.

"No problems we didn't take care of," they told him.

"Good. I'll see ya all later."

"Won't ya come in Julie?" Weld invited.

"Yes, I have some things to discuss with Gladys."

Inside, there was no sign of Gladys.

"She must be down around the barn or the chicken house." Weld stated. "Fill me in on everything that has been going on since I left."

"I don't know much about the ranch or its workings," Julie told him. "However Gladys did say that everything was going just like clockwork that the hands all worked well together and accomplished good results."

"Ya can't ask fer anything better than that," Weld opined.

Weld said tentatively, "I was rather surprised when Bob returned home, saying he was there fer good. I thought maybe the two of ya had a thing going."

"No, we were just friends. No romance of any kind. However I do think Bob might have misinterpreted somewhat so I told him a little white lie. I told him I was engaged. I didn't want to lead him on."

"Julie, so's there will be no misunderstanding between us, I'd like ta say the first time I saw ya I wanted ta ask ya out. I found my brother Bob was interested in ya, so I backed off. Is there any chance ya might consent ta see me in a definite romantic way?"

"I waited over a year for you to just notice me," Julie admitted. "I'd like very much to see you as often as you wish."

He took a step toward her just as he heard the backdoor open and stopped as Gladys came into the room. "Weld!" she cried, hugging him tightly "I didn't know you were returning for a while yet. How are you?"

"I'm fine," he told her, "a bit frazzled, but a good night's sleep will fix that up."

"Hello Julie. Did you come for the produce?"

"No, but I'll be glad to pick up all you have. I always feel better and rest better after I've been here. I've always loved the country."

Julie glanced at Weld saying, "later perhaps." As she followed Gladys out the door to get food for the homeless. Weld nodded.

There was much talk of Weld's travels and all he had seen. Then they caught up on the ranch business and gossip. "Did they get the load of cattle from the fall roundup picked up at the junction? How much did they clear?" Etc.

Weld hit the sack about seven thirty, just after supper and slept until noon the next day. No one even attempted to wake him.

Julie was eager to be alone with Weld to discuss their feelings for each other but she had to wait for him to make the first move. "A woman never being able to openly pursue a man wasn't fair." Julie stormed to herself. Why should it make a difference if she were to let everyone know she wanted Weld badly? Why should she or any other woman end up a tarnished woman with talk of being a whore for being the aggressor?

There! She said it. Whore! Whore! It wasn't that she was a virgin she definitely was not. It was more or less accepted in her social circle that girls eighteen or over had flirtations with physical contact, maybe with several different young men. She had gone steady for six months with Dwight Hall when she was seventeen and eighteen. They hade made love or at least had sex. She had never liked it. She just let Dwight do it because he wanted to. However when she just thought of Weld she had urges she had never before experienced. She longed to have him kiss her and hold her close. "Ohhh my!" she despaired.

Weld was kept busy for several days rounding up the cattle that were calving right then to protect the newborn calves from wolves and coyotes. They also had some bobcats that preyed on the baby animals. The cows had a habit of going into a gully to have their young so they didn't have to search the entire ranch. However some of the animals did stay with the herds and dropped their calves there.

It was spring and time to weed out every non-layer, crippled, injured or otherwise not a producer and take them to market. The hens were grouchy grumbling like a pregnant woman does sometimes, wanting to set. Eggs had to be placed in nests for them.

Usually twenty to thirty hens were setting at once on twelve to sixteen eggs each. A new batch would be set after twenty one days. Weld loved to see the baby chickens with the mama chickens scratching and clucking to her brood. When a shower would come up the mama hens would cluck furiously spreading their wings to cover their babies. "There just ain't nothin' like a mother's love," Weld said aloud as he saw a hen hovering a brood that was maybe three weeks old.

They culled out fifty of the hogs that weighed approximately one hundred fifty pounds each to take to market. Next month, there would be another fifty or so. New piglets were being born every day now. About two thirds of the beef cattle would go to market this spring roundup which would start next week, Weld reckoned. During spring roundup it was very busy because that is also planting time for corn, oats and hay. They would need six more hands during that time.

The horses would also be taken to sell off, leaving only brood stock and colts. In late fall they would roundup, brand and sell again. Just after fall roundup was the time of least work but they still had plenty to do. Everything from fence mending to repairing saddles and bridles had to be done and ready for busy times. Boards, doors, floors, haylofts, pigpens, chicken roosts, wood for making new stalls and for heating and cooking had to be gathered and stored for repair work. Spring and early summer was food, preserving time as well. Two thousand quarts of fruits and vegetables would be canned. Corn would be dried or canned, or shelled for the animals. It was run through the coarse grinder to make chicken feed and left on the ear for pigs and horses. Jerky was dried and meat was canned at any butchering time.

Weld took off for town Friday night, telling the boys to look for him when they saw him coming. “I may stay in town tonight.”

He hoped to see Julie, but if he couldn’t he would visit Big Bertha’s place. He knew a couple of sweet girls there unless they had left while he was gone.

He found Julie her hands deep in dishwater at the soup kitchen. “What are ya doin’ dishes fer? There is a room full of people out there that would be glad ta help out with the dishwashing I’ll bet.”

He went into the hall and pointed to a couple of young men, maybe twenty five or six to follow him. “We need some help in here with the dishes. Would one of ya wash and the other dry please?” he smiled.

“Sure, glad to,” one of them said and the other nodded.

“Woman, come with me.” Weld said.

“Gladly, O Master! “she whispered.

She could not leave her car unattended, so she drove her car and Weld followed in Black Beauty. Julie invited Weld into her apartment she kept downtown in San Francisco. “Be seated Weld, I’ll be right back," she said as she disappeared into her bedroom. Shortly she reentered the parlor her hair let down, hanging to her waist. She had a tray in her hands with tall glasses of milk and a plate of homemade cookies. She placed the tray on the table in front of the settee. Weld took the milk but ignored the cookies. He held her hand as she held the cookie plate toward him.

"I'm not hungry for food, only for ya." Weld told her. "I have been attracted ta ya, dreaming of ya and needin' ya since that first day. May I kiss ya?" he asked.

"Please do. I've imagined kissing you for so long. Wait Weld, I want to tell you, I'm no virgin."

"Neither am I," Weld laughed, "I haven't been since I was sixteen."

"You are a man. It doesn't matter for a man so I just wanted to be up front with you all the way."

"Will ya just shut up and come here?" he asked as he pulled her to her feet, holding her tenderly kissing her softly.

This was a whole new experience for Weld. He wanted to protect her even from herself. He didn't press himself into her but held her softly away.

"Why?" she asked when he put her from him.

"Julie, ya are not just a lay in the hay fer me. Ya are what we cowhands call prime stuff. and ya don't mishandle prime stuff," he told her.

"Umm!" she said. I have no such feelings. I mix my life everyday with those I help and serve. I'm not easily breakable. My self-image is intact. My body is longing for you and I intend to have you now, right here." She demanded, "Come!"

Weld said, "are ya absolutely sure?"

"I'm more than sure."

Hours later Weld pondered just what his feelings were for Julie. He certainly cared for her but he just didn't know how deep that feeling was. He had thought he cared more deeply for her before, but!! Maybe it was because Julie really doesn't need anything that he felt strangely about her. She has everything already. She responded to his lovemaking but offered little in return. He wasn't even sure if she even felt anything. Nooo, he just didn't know about her.

Julie felt herself wondering along those same lines. She was so sure that she loved Weld and would marry him. He had made love to her in everyway possible but she just didn't feel much. "I think I'm frigid!"

Weld was picking up freight at the depot when he saw Dottie. "Hello." He said more cheerily than he felt. "Did ya get married?" he asked.

"No I did not. I was waiting for you to come back and carry me off, but you didn't show up," she snapped.

"But ya told me ya were getting married!" he said plaintively.

"Why didn't you know I was just trying to make you jealous?" she cried with real tears in her pretty eyes. "I've just been miserable," she pouted. "I've watched for you everyplace. Why can't you love me as I do you?" she demanded.

Weld was stunned. He realized he did love her. He probably had from the first. He held out his arms and she ran into them. "In this public place, someone will see us," she said.

"Let them. We don't care." Weld said as he kissed her thoroughly. "We will come back later for our freight." he told the clerk, rushing Dottie toward her apartment.

As soon as they entered the doorway, Dottie demanded of Weld, "hold me, kiss me, love me," as she was trying to get out of her clothes and at the same time pulling at his.

"Baby, baby, I've missed ya. I've tried ta deny it ta myself, but I couldn't. As I slept I dreamed of making love ta ya. I could see yer sweet face everywhere."

She punched him hard. "Why did you make me suffer? You, you fake." she sobbed. "I wanted to die. I wanted to kill you. I still may. I might just love you to death."

"Give it a try, what a wonderful way ta go."

She tried, they never did light the lamp in the parlor.

****

CHAPTER 24

Jackson and Henry landed in New York, May 15th, 1915. They had been working for the railroad all over the west for the last few months. Jack had gotten to run the engine for thirty miles. The engineer took a liking to Jack and let him handle the engine just for fun.

They had worked beside those small men from China. They were small, but they did twice the work the other men did and received less pay. They were also preyed upon and mistreated by fellow workers. Both Jack and Henry had banged around on some fellers for banging around on the little men.

"It's time we tried our hand at some kind of sea vessel," Jack said. Here they were, tired and dirty, looking for a place to bathe, change clothes and sleep. In the morning they would check into either working on a ship, or buying a ticket to London. They had decided to visit Jenny, one way or another. They had all the information as to where she had her business and where she lived. They wouldn't stay long. They just wanted the adventure. Maybe they would go to Paris and see Lizzet and Weld's sculpture as well. They were a pair of happy boys.

"We better wait a day or so before we go." Henry said. "We need ta visit all the art galleries and museums here. I'd like ta go up in some of those tall buildings too.

"All right, we need ta go ta a bank ta cash a check ta travel on anyway," Jack said. "Ya got your bank letter and identification Henry?"

"Yep! I got everything I'm supposed ta have I reckon."

"Look at those gals over there with that short hair and all that paint on their faces." Henry pointed. "Look how short their dresses are. Ya can see halfway up ta their knees."

"What would mama say ta that?" Jack snorted.

They walked for what seemed miles, gawking at everything and looking for their bank. People jostled into them, not even saying, "Sorry."

Jack thought they should buy some new clothes to travel in cause they sure weren't dressed like anyone here. They passed many stores with dummies dressed like people. They finally stopped at one, getting fitted out in the latest dress mode, according to the clerk.

"Well, latest mode maybe, but I ain't wearing that tie or that silly looking hat," Henry stated.

"And neither am I," Jack echoed.

Now they looked just like everyone else on the street but they weren't sure they wanted to look like everyone else. They did notice they got better service now and people weren't pointing and snickering at them.

"Ya know people here ain't very nice." Jack said. "They don't seem ta have any manners."

"Well, we won't be here very long. Just pretend not ta hear," Henry suggested.

They had to purchase tickets to London and the accommodations weren't too wonderful but the boys were having a great time. Neither of them became seasick. There were a group of young ladies on board chaperoned by a stern looking silver haired woman. She tried to keep her girls away from the other passengers but youth will find a way. Every afternoon Midge Welch took a nap on deck. She left the girls on their honor not to do anything that would make her sorry she had agreed to watch over them en route to an all girl's school in London. All the girls and most of the single males gathered on the opposite side of the ship out of sight of Miz Welch to have fun. Some of them sang, some of the boys played French harps and some of them danced. Anytime, anywhere a Winter heard music, they danced. It gave them a chance to have names and school addresses when they reached London.

Jack met a small girl of about seventeen. She was very pretty, petite, friendly and loved to dance. Her name was Cindy.

Miz Welch never did catch any of them. Shipboard romances happened every trip, one girl informed Henry but they usually did not last past docking. Henry was hoping that was the way of it with Jack, but Jack sure was smitten with Cindy and if Henry was any judge of it, Cindy felt the same way about Jack.

Henry liked all girls, but that was all, just liked. He had always wondered if he would even marry. He knew one thing. He did not want a wife or anyone else trying to run his life. He might or might not want to do something good or bad, but no one else was going to make up his mind for him.

He thought he might open a small business or even a fix it shop. He had always been good with his hands. When he was twelve he made a saddle and it was a good one.

It lasted him until he grew out of it. Now it was at the farm for the younguns to use. He made a beautiful bridle with silver adornments. It was the one Weld used most when he was home. Henry could build buildings and plain furniture and toys as well. He made the girls buggies for their dolls and playhouses too. "Yep!" he thought. "I just think I might do that."

It was a sad time for the new found friends the night before docking. Henry saw Jack holding Cindy, kissing her over and over. They both looked sad.

Everyone smiled through tears, bidding good-bye to everyone else.

Henry was already looking for a driver while Jack was still watching Cindy being herded into one of the waiting automobiles. He loaded up his and Jack's stuff calling to Jack to hurry. Finally Jack crawled in beside him. Henry had already shown the address to the driver and they were on their way. Henry was wide eyed over everything but Jack sat in silence. His mind was on how he was ever going to get to see Cindy again.

It seemed as if they had just started when the driver parked outside the huge doors to the Arlton castle. They had been told of the size, the look and all but nothing they had heard had prepared them for this.

The liveried doorman, said, "May I ask who is calling sirs?"

"Yes, we are Jenny's brothers, Jack and Henry."

"This way please." Opening the great door, he announced "Mr. Jack and Henry Winter to see Miz Jenny."

A man carrying a young boy came to greet them. "I am Jenny's husband James, and this," he pointed to the child, "is James Jacob, your nephew. Do come in. Jenny will be home in a short time.

She seldom goes into the shop these days but today there was some kind of problem."

"I'm so sorry for your loss. I liked both Jacob and Abby very much," James said.

"Thank ya." Jack said. "We are finally dealing with it. It takes a long time. Pardon me James, but would ya mind if I just stood here and stared? I know it's very unsophisticated, but I'm just a country boy. I've never seen such…such."

"Opulence?" James said.

"Yes! That's the word."

"Well, don't be overpowered by it. It's just stuff, it's not what is really important in life. I really never even notice it."

"Papa said ya were just a good ol' boy wrapped in gold cloth. He was right. He also said Jenny was so fortunate to have fallen in love with a real man."

"That means a lot to me," James said. "Thank you for telling me.

They moved on to Jenny and James' apartment inside the castle.

"A feller could get lost in here and never be seen again," Jack laughed.

James pulled the servants cord and asked them to bring milk and ham sandwiches for the boys and some of that cream pie that was left.

In just a very few minutes a maid returned with a tray of sandwiches and tall glasses of milk. The pie looked good.

James watched Henry and Jack eating as if it were their last meal. All of the Winter men were voracious eaters and never gained an ounce.

The kitchen help were told the Winter boys were here so to remember what kind of foods they liked and to serve them at least twice the size of normal portions.

"How is Weld?" James inquired.

"Well, he went back to California ta the Bar-X-Z. They are probably plenty busy right about now. This is a busy season fer ranchers and farmers," Jack informed James.

"Oh! Farmers and ranchers are different?" James queried.

"Farms usually grow crops of feed grains and vegetables, fruit, eggs milk and that sort of thing. On the other hand ranchers mostly raise cattle, horses, hogs, plus they raise a lot of hay and corn ta feed the animals through the winter. I understand California where Weld is, has pasture year 'round, but they still raise a lot of hay and corn. I think ranching is better, because of the full time planting, growing and harvesting that a farm requires. If ya have a thousand acres, ya can move the cattle from pasture ta pasture, while the first one is growing again and then move them back again. Cattle do not spoil if it is too rainy or if left in the field too long. Produce has to done at exactly the right time or ya will lose your britches."

"My what?" James inquired.

"Oh ya know, your tail and all its fixtures, your trousers, your pants."

"Oh yes, I remember now. Jacob called it your ass and all its fixtures," he laughed.

Jenny nearly fainted when she saw both boys relaxing with James and baby. "Where did you come from? My goodness how you have grown, you were babies when I last saw you. Is it four or five years now?" she exclaimed. I'm so glad to see you. Who would have thought it would have been you younguns that would come here? How was your trip? Were you seasick?"

"We had a grand time all the way over. We met some young ladies on board sang and danced a little and no we did not get sick, but plenty of folks did," Henry laughed.

Jack asked about girl's schools where they were located and such?

"There are many schools for girls all over London. Are you looking for anyone special?" James asked.

"Yes, this one." Showing the name and address on the paper Cindy had written on.

"Oh that's just across the way," he said, pointing toward the north. It is maybe three quarters of a mile, a little more or a little less," he explained. "You can walk or ride one of their horses right up to their fence. I don't know if you could get close enough to speak to anyone but you could try."

Jack rose and shook James' hand. It was the first real smile he had shown since they had arrived.

Now that Jack had loosened up he was full of nonsense putting Jenny in mind of Weld. He had a quick wit and that same secret little smile Weld carried around with him. The one that made the girls swoon.

James gave the boys an Arlton's card that would get them in any place and pay for anything they purchased.

"What a deal!" Henry said. "Ya mean all I have ta do is show this card and doors will open fer me?"

Jenny laughed and assured him that was the case. "How old are you now Henry?" Jenny asked.

"I'll soon be 23," he said.

"How old are you now Jack?" she probed.

"I'm 24, I'll be twenty five in eight months."

They seemed so young to be traveling around but then she remembered she was only eighteen when she left home.

"Ya know we talked about goin' ta Paris to see that Can-Can dance Mama and Papa went ta see and the statue of Weld at that hotel," Henry informed her. I hear there are a lot of things ta see and do in Paris. We would like ta meet Lizzet, who painted mama and sculpted Weld. Do ya think she will see us?'

"Oh I'm sure she would. From what Weld and Mama and Papa said, she is very nice.

"Jack ain't goin' anyplace until he figures out how ta see that girl again." Henry complained. "I may hafta go by myself. Have ya met Lizzet or seen the statue yet?"

"No, we haven't. We have discussed it, but just haven't done it yet," admitted Jenny.

"Maybe we can all go." Henry suggested.

"Umm, I don't know. I'll speak to James about it.

"Jenny, if Jack can't see or speak ta that Cindy Smythe, do ya suppose ya might be able ta invite her fer a weekend or something? Jack's a good feller. He would never do anything ta harm Cindy or any good girl. He really is a gentleman."

"I don't know but I'll ask Peggy. She knows everyone and I doubt is anyone would turn down an invitation from an Arlton."

Jack and Henry went into town, driven by Arlton's chauffer. He took them all over London, including the girl's school where Cindy went and lived in one of the dormitories where they stayed two girls to a room. Jack's eyes strained to see Cindy but no one was outside at that time. Jack felt better just seeing where she was.

Henry didn't mention that Jenny was checking with Peggy to see if they could invite Cindy to the castle for a weekend. "No use getting Jack's hopes up, just in case."

They had sent letters home and one to Weld just before they had left New York, saying where they would be for awhile. When the mail came they had letters from Bob and the family and from Weld as well. All of them were giving them advice about what to do, like always. At least it showed they all cared.

Jenny received a letter from the family too asking her to keep an eye on the boys. “They are rowdy and could get into trouble they can’t get out of,” the family worried.

James told the boys they could all go tho Paris just as soon as the next ship embarked for there. If they still wanted to go he would book passage for all of them.

Jack looked forlorn. He really wanted to go to Paris he just wanted to see Cindy if possible.

Jenny told Jack, “Peggy is working on being able to invite Cindy for a weekend, but it could not happen for a couple or three or maybe more, weeks. She had to wire Cindy’s folks to get permission before the school will allow her to go anyplace. This is a good thing. They are protecting the girls.”

Jack was so excited and happy that he might see Cindy but sad it would take so long. He was ready to go to Paris.

It was just a short distance to Paris but time seemed to pass slowly. James got a little sick but soon got over it.

James had made all the reservations and had arranged for two drivers of conveyance to meet them at the dock and to be at their disposal while they were there.

The first thing all of them all of them wanted to do was to see the sculpture of Weld, then on to Lizzet's. That's just what they did. They went first to the hotel where they would be staying then to the hotel where the statue was displayed. Many people were there looking at all of the artwork that was on display but the piece they all like best was Weld.

"It is a beautiful thing," Jenny proposed. "It looks just like him. There is that little smile and that little scar on his back where he slipped and cut himself at about sixteen years of age."

"Look everyone! Here he is. He is the one. Lizzet's work!" They said, looking at Jack.

"No, No, that's not me. That's my brother. I don't pose."

"He's your brother? Where is he? We want to meet him."

"He is in America, California. He will be pleased to know you admire him."

Henry and Jack had seen the miniature sculpture Lizzet had sent to Abby and Jacob, but a life size, of every part of your body, nude. Well Henry would certainly never pose for one like that.

Jack said, "I don't know, it might be fun. I think it is a beautiful piece of art."

Henry just shook his head. He was amazed Jack could even consider such a thing.

When they reached Lizzet's, Jenny and James led the way and knocked at her studio door.

"Entre vous." Lizzet said in French. Only James understood French.

"Can we speak English please?" James asked.

"But of course we can. How may I help you?" she inquired.

She glanced up seeing Jack. She rose putting her arms around Jack, kissing his cheek. "Weld, I am so happy to see you. Have you come to pose for me again?" Then she looked at him more closely.

"Oh you are not Weld. I am so sorry. You must be his brother. You look almost exactly like him. Are you his sister Jenny and her husband James? Now who might you be?" she asked Henry. You must be a brother as well. You have that same look, only a little more like Abby. Does she like the portrait and the miniature of Weld? Is Jacob pleased with them?"

Jenny said, "My mother and father are both dead. They died within fourteen hours of each other."

"My God! This cannot be. They were strong healthy people, very much in love. When? How?"

Jenny explained what had happened. "Mama just lay down and died not being able to face life without Papa."

"Yes, they must be together for all time. A love like theirs can do no less," Lizzet declared. "Are you here for a holiday or have you come to stay for some time?"

"Just a couple of days are all we can free up just now," Jenny said.

"Jack, can we talk for a few minutes?" Lizzet asked.

"Certainly!" Jack said.

"Please let me sketch you and take measurements. I know your sister cannot stay, but can you? I am inspired by Winter men and your mother as well. I made a smaller portrait of your mother as I painted the large canvas. I would give it to you if you would sit for me."

"How long would I have ta pose?"

"One week, then off two days, then back for perhaps four days. I then would need you off and on for a week while I get the wire frame just right and each muscle measured so I can start building the entire work. Two months total."

"I can't be away from Jenny's that long. We have something planned."

"Can't you go back for whatever it is then come back here for awhile?"

"Well, I'll ask Jenny how we might work it out."

Jenny agreed that he could stay for maybe three weeks before there might be a chance to see Cindy. He could then go back to London for a few days before crossing back again. She thought it could be worked out.

Jack would stay but Henry would return to London.

When Lizzet and Jack had gotten to work, Lizzet told Jack to strip. He did it as if he had been doing it all of his life in front of a stranger, a woman.

Lizzet turned his head, feeling the skull shape with nimble fingers, then down his arms hefting them to feel just where the muscles wrapped across. She was as impersonal as someone buying a horse. Probing, sighting, she ran her fingers all down his back, all over his chest, over his buttocks and down his thighs, skipping, Sam. If she had shown one personal act, he would have been gone but she didn't. Weld had never told him or anyone of the lovemaking after the project was finished.

Jenny had given him and Henry the names and addresses of the people and places Weld had visited but he could find his own friends or not, as he wished.

Jack visited dozens of places of interest driven by Lizzet's driver. Jack invited the driver to accompany him because he liked company and because he could not speak or understand French. He needed to know the history of the things he saw and the driver supplied him with that. He went back to see Weld's sculpture examining it thoroughly. "Don't look now brother dear but I'm gonna be standing right next ta ya and I'm gonna be PURDIER," he laughed.

Foster, Lizzet's driver took Jack to the same clubs Weld visited. Jack saw the same tall dark woman with the deep eyes as Weld had. He was taken to her room and made love to by her as he made love to her just as Weld had with all the sweet words, tender touches and loveing technique. She enjoyed him much as she had Weld. There was so little difference in Weld and Jack they were almost as the same person.

Jack joined the musicians playing the fiddle, making it wail sadly then happily. He loved music all kinds of music.

He felt no infidelity to Cindy. Ladies of the night are a panacea for single men until they married.

Jack was about finished posing for Lizzet. The sculpture had already become a full, bodied head finished sculpture. Jack had posed in the opposite direction of Weld. He was also more frontal with a twist of the torso. It was beautiful and Lizzet made a smaller piece for Jack to take home with him along with his portrait of his mother.

Lizzet did not make any move toward Jack. No loving, no nothing, except a hug and many thanks that he had stayed to let her finish to the point she did not need Jack now.

Back in London, Jenny had good news for Jack. Peggy was having a small gathering next Saturday. She had invited several of her friend's young members of their families as well as Cindy, who had been given permission to attend.

Jack was excited but maybe a little less than before he went to Paris. Somehow he had grown emotionally as a man, an adult. He still wanted to see Cindy but he would not die if he did not.

There were half dozen beautiful, young ladies beside Cindy at the gathering. There was plenty of music, dancing and food. Jack danced with Cindy and with every other girl there. Henry on the other hand danced little and preferred to watch than to participate. He had a great time. He just had a different way of enjoying himself.

Jenny watched from a distance. She watched Jack carefully. She had been worried about Jack's infatuation with Cindy. Now she could see everything would be all right. The Winter boys were a strong bunch. They were level headed not easy to intimidate, physically or emotionally. They were all gentlemen, never taking advantage of anyone, male or female. Jenny thought Papa and Mama could be proud of all their children, even her.

Henry was ready to go back to America. He had seen and done wonderful things, but there was no place like home.

Jack hadn't decided what he wanted to do yet. He was visiting factories and manufacturing places, learning how everything worked. Jenny's Place of Design, fascinated him to see a piece of material go from a sketch to a finished garment was amazing. There were dozens of women and several men running those fast sewing machines. How quickly the cutters finished a total pattern then it went on to the next step.

He thought "I'd like to do this and I bet I could too."

James explained every step of the business procedure from Arlton's, or Jenny's conception through every cost of every scrap of paper or needle.

Henry left for America two and a half months of his arrival back in London from Paris. Jack did not go back. He had fallen in love with England, deciding to stay at least a year to see what he really wanted to do.

James encouraged Jack to start out at once learning the business. He really liked Jack and saw that he had great potential in the business end of Jenny's as well as Arlton's. He was like a sponge soaking up information and suggesting how things might be improved upon.

****

CHAPTER 25

Weld and Dottie announced their engagement to the people at the Bar-X-Z at a roundup dance. Everyone was taken by surprise. No one had even heard him speak of Dottie here to fore. Everyone wished them happiness.

“When is the big day?” Gladys asked.

“We haven’t decided yet, but soon.” Weld answered.

Dottie was a beautiful woman and it was plain to see they were crazy for each other. No one had ever seen Weld so openly attentive to any woman. He always kept his private life, very private.

Telegrams were sent to family members, advising of the coming nuptials.

No one could come just now. Everything had been realigned at the farm. The married folk had their hands full with crops and animals. It was school time for the girls, but they were all very happy for Weld. They said they had not believed he would ever settle down. Etc.

The wedding was a beautiful affair. There were lots of friends dancing and the eating of good foods, singing and just having a good time.

Weld was happier than he had ever been and to think he had almost lost her. "He had always been lucky," he smiled to himself.

Dottie had never believed that Weld would ever marry her. Now that he had she had a secret to admit to. On their wedding night she told him she had lied to him the very first night she had met him. "I told you that I could not have children, but I can. I just know the salty egg remedy to keep from getting pregnant," she told him.

"What is the salty egg remedy?" he asked her.

"Simply to insert salt, into the vagina, in a capsule or from a tube. A salty egg will not hatch," she smiled.

"Well, no more salty eggs. We need to get started at once working on a family. That was the only fly in the ointment I had in wanting ta marry ya. I come from a big family of twelve. I love children but half that number is fine," he said as he expertly undressed her.

They would spend part of their time at the ranch and part of it at Dottie's apartment. He had no intention of asking her to stop working.

She would have to decide that on her own. His life was wonderful, he was happy.

****

CHAPTER 26

Henry arrived at the ranch with no previous announcement.

"Where is Jack?" Everyone wanted to know. "Is he visiting someone in town before he comes home?"

"Nope! He ain't in town and he won't be coming home fer awhile. He decided to stay in London with Jenny. He likes the place. I don't see how, but he does. He also is very interested in clothing manufacturing and is working for Jenny and Arlton's. He is fine, very content, happy."

Bob had changed a few things in the running of the ranch. Since the boys had so much to attend to for themselves they did not want to stay on at the farm. They would be working only at roundup and at harvest as extra hands after selling their shares of the farm to Bob.

An extra room addition was made for the hands to have their meals in. Bob felt it was better to keep the help from the young girls while they were growing up. Sometimes, some hands are a little rough around the edges. Also Raye wanted to start a family right away not leaving a lot of extra room to have the hands in the house. Everyone was happy with their place in the family knowing where and what their part was in the household.

Bob had met Gloria Wister at a dance. They were engaged to be married in December at Christmas time. She was beautiful and as well adjusted a young woman as Bob was a man. Life was great.

Frank and Margie were expecting. Jerry and Carly already had a new baby boy. Carl and Pansy were not pregnant yet but you could not tell about those Winter boys.

Henry has his little business started with more work than he could handle. He was thinking of hiring a helper. He had kept his share in the farm. He had spent less than half his cash in traveling and opening up the shop. He still didn't think marriage was for him, and unlike his brothers and sisters he knew darned well he didn't want any younguns. He had always felt crowded with so many folks in the house.

Raye and Bob say Abby and Jacob are everywhere in the house. They often imagined them sitting in the parlor looking at Abby's portrait. They could see Jacob holding Abby's hand leaning their heads together not talking. They had not seemed to need words.

****

CHAPTER 27

Julie found solace in her work, but just wasn't interested in looking for romance. She and Gladys continued to help feed, house, clothe, school and medicate those in need.

Gillie returned home from England. She had hoped to snare a rich man of title but she just couldn't pretend to enjoy sex. She had experimented with various fellows hoping to find someone she could at least stand to be with, but to no avail. She hated the touch of any man who came near her.

Weld had married, Bob had gone back to Kansas and had taken over the Winter Farm so Gilly knew very few men in or around San Francisco. Those she did know were poor and Gilly certainly would not entertain the idea of a poor man. She now had money of her own but she was not about to take care of some slob of a cowpoke.

Gilly's mother Gladys was still cool toward her, but Gilly didn't give a hoot about that either. Now that she was of age she would do as she darned well felt like.

Gladys had gotten Gilly to go along with her to the soup kitchens. Although she did not feel compassion for these folks as her mother did, Gilly enjoyed getting out of the house and away from cattle and all talk about ranching. Another thing, she did not like eating at the table with hired help. Weld and Dottie were always underfoot and so were Jake and Slade. Oh she knew her father had left Weld a one third interest in the ranch, as well as other income but as far as she was concerned, he was just hired help and so was his wife.

Gilly was thinking about getting herself a place in town. She could at least choose the people she fraternized with.

Gilly met Julie her second week back from abroad. They hit it off really well. Julie was no country bumpkin. Gilly got so tired of country slang and accents. At least in England people had good manners and could speak of something other than horses and cows.

Julie invited Gilly to spend the weekend at her home away from the city. Gilly accepted right away. She could envision a lavish mansion where the smell of horseflesh did not permeate everything.

Julie had made arrangements for them to go to the theater that evening and to the cinema to see a movie the next day that they had both professed the desire to see.

After the theater they dined in a fantastic restaurant. The food and the service were wonderful. Soft music played somewhere in the background soothing their nerves. Both of them were mellow and relaxed.

As they left the restaurant, Julie's hand touched Gilly's side, sending an electrical shock through the both of them. Julie looked at Gilly questioningly. Gilly was stunned. She was searching her brain for an answer. All she knew was she wanted Julie to touch her again, plus more. She really didn't know what more, she was confused. Julie felt the same way. She had a strong urge to kiss Gilly. She was astonished. Why should she want to kiss a woman, any woman?

Their driver picked them up and delivered them back home. Once inside, they just stood looking at each other, neither knowing what to think or do. Finally Julie took Gilly's hand and led her upstairs. Entering Julie's huge bedroom they locked the door.

Gilly stood stock still, but Julie began undoing Gilly's dress, letting it fall to the floor. She then pulled Gilly's slip up over her head and bent to kiss Gilly's lips, both of them gasping, holding on to each other. Gilly and Julie hurriedly got Julie's clothes off, then with both stripped naked they began touching each other in wonder.

"What is, is this?" Gilly whispered.

"I don't know," Julie said, "but I want to touch you and kiss you."

"Me too," Gilly answered.

Gilly moved in with Julie. They both blossomed and everyone commented on how healthy and happy they looked. Both of them worked very hard trying to do for the poor children. Even Gilly had begun to feel real compassion for those who came to the soup kitchens with the little children with the sad eyes.

Julie took over Gilly's life. She made her decisions for her and told her what to do and how to feel. Gilly loved it. She loved pleasing Julie and was so glad she would never have to have children. She had never wanted children but knew a man would always want babies. It is part of their genetic make up. Somehow babies proved a man's manhood. "Silly!" she thought.

Julie never wanted children either. She saw too much sadness surrounding helpless little waifs. Any mothering she needed to do would be satisfied helping the poor families of the streets.

Someday Julie and Gilly would let the world in on their love but for now, they just enjoyed their lives together.

CHAPTER 28

In the end, some of the siblings used the cash they had inherited to buy the other's shares of the farm.

There were and still are strong love matches, romances and dalliances by the Winter men, but always as gentlemen.

The farm is still in the Winter family where the influence of Jacob and Abby Winter's strong family creed still guide the new generations.

Weld sired two sons that each went into politics. The eldest became an aide to the Governer and went on to become a diplomat to a small country in Asia.

The youngest boy became a liason to the president.

Weld's daughter went to London, becoming a designer for Arlton's.

Bob fathered five boys. All but one of them stayed on the farm until they married and had farms of their own. Bob's youngest son had his Dad's itchy feet and a love for the law, which he settled into at twenty five years of age.

All of the brothers except Henry, married and raised large families. Henry never married but became a very good businessman, making a very good living from the five stores he owned.

Jack didn't marry until he was forty one. He always said, "I can't find anyone that will have me."

Of course, the ladies pursued him as they had all those Winter boys, until Peggy White roped him and hogtied him for life.

~FINI~

ABOUT THE AUTHOR

Lola Elizabeth Neeley, born December twenty third, nineteen twenty five, in Oklahoma became a first time author at seventy five.

She is one of eight children and a mother of four. She has three daughters, Carolyn, Lacquanna and Victoria. Her one son, Billy was killed in a motorcycle accident in nineteen seventy-four.

Printed in the United States
134568LV00001B/50/A

9 781410 747396